Nurses in the Political Arena

The Public Face of Nursing

Harriet R. Feldman, PhD, RN, FAAN, is Dean and Professor of Nursing at Pace University Lienhard School of Nursing in New York. She is editor of *Nursing Leadership Forum,* published by Springer Publishing Company. She has been politically active in nursing, holding a number of leadership positions in the New York State Nurses Association, American Association of Colleges of Nursing, and statewide deans' organizations in New York and New Jersey. Her interests in the political activities of nurses and their involvement in shaping public policy have grown through these leadership positions and through her role as member of the American Nurses Association House of Delegates. Dr. Feldman is a noted author of more than 60 scholarly publications, including books, book chapters, journal articles, and editorials, and has presented at national and international conferences. She received her PhD from New York University and her MS and BS degrees from Adelphi University. She also has a certificate from the Management Development Program at Harvard University.

Sandra B. Lewenson, EdD, RN, is Professor of Nursing and Associate Dean for Academic Affairs at Pace University Lienhard School of Nursing in New York. Prior to her appointment at Pace University, Dr. Lewenson served as the Director of Accreditation at the National League for Nursing. Her interest in the political activities of nurses and nursing spans the late 19th and 20th centuries. Her research has focused on nursing's involvement in the women's suffrage movement at the beginning of the 20th century and has provided the basis for her work on exploring how nursing is valued in society. She is the author of several books, articles, and videos about nursing's political involvement and activism. In 1995 her book, *Taking Charge: Nursing, Suffrage, and Feminism 1873–1920* won the prestigious American Association for the History of Nursing, Lavinia Dock Award for Historical Scholarship and Research in Nursing. Dr. Lewenson received her EdD and MEd from Teachers College, Columbia University, her MS from Mercy College, and BS from Hunter College.

Nurses in the Political Arena

The Public Face of Nursing

Harriet R. Feldman, PhD, RN, FAAN
Sandra B. Lewenson, EdD, RN

SP SPRINGER PUBLISHING COMPANY

Springer Publishing Company, Inc.
536 Broadway
New York, NY 10012-3955

Acquisitions Editor: Sheri W. Sussman
Production Editor: Pamela Lankas
Cover design by Susan Hauley

00 01 02 03 04 / 5 4 3 2 1

Library of Congress Cataloging-in-Publication Data

Feldman, Harriet R.
    Nurses in the political arena : the public face of nursing / Harriet R.
  Feldman and Sandra B. Lewenson
       p. cm.
    Includes bibliographical references and index.
    ISBN 0-8261-1331-1
    1. Nursing—Political aspects.   2. Nursing—Social aspects.
  3. Nurses—Interviews.   I. Lewenson, Sandra. II. Title.
RT86.5 .F45 2000
362.1′73—dc21
                                                      00-030090

Printed in the United States of America

Contents

Acknowledgments

No effort worth doing is done alone. For us, writing this book was a community effort—colleagues, new friends, and our families joined us in telling the stories of success and challenge that needed to be told. We believe, as do many of those we interviewed, that these stories can serve to both mentor others and to promote the betterment of society.

Colleagues from Pace University listened to our ideas and helped us to crystallize the themes that emerged from the interviews. The Hot Logs research group of the Lienhard School of Nursing helped to identify initial themes, and Karen Anderson Keith read the manuscript and offered her insights on both content and form.

Our graduate assistant, Lisette Barton, greatly facilitated our work by providing the structure that led us to the interviews, as well as the literature and electronic searches, assistance with the appendices, and follow-up on just about anything we asked. Even with all the work we assigned to her as a graduate assistant, Lizette asked to do more and more on the project because of her growing interest in the topic.

The people we interviewed became "new friends," as they helped us to understand their experiences, hopes, concerns, and admonitions. Each one contributed his or her ideas openly and freely and made us feel that our work was right "on target."

Our husbands, Ron Feldman and Richard Lewenson, gave us input, criticism, and lots of support through the many hours and days, and some very late nights, as together and separately we wrote and critiqued, then wrote some more. Our children, Craig and Jaime Feldman and Jennifer and Nicole Lewenson, all recent college graduates, added their encouragement and thoughts.

We particularly want to acknowledge the foresight and unconditional support of Dr. Ursula Springer; this, together with Sheri

Sussman's thoughtful approach to working with authors and patience in getting books to press, was very much appreciated.

Last, we want to acknowledge the colleagueship and true sharing between us as well as the humor and openness that became the highlights of our work together.

HARRIET R. FELDMAN, PHD, RN, FAAN
SANDRA B. LEWENSON, EDD, RN

Foreword

Why encourage nurses to run for public office? What makes it important—or what makes a nurse a special case over any other woman or man who has the "fire in the belly" to take on this daunting challenge? Does it matter to those of us who are nurses, and why? Does it matter to the general public? My answer to the last two questions is an unequivocal "yes," and this answer suggests the answers to the first two questions.

When I heard about this book, these questions were the ones I needed to answer for myself to determine how important I thought the book was. I have asked and answered the same questions as I have worked with colleagues across the country and watched them and other nurses move into the policy arena and particularly that involved with running for office. How can nurses make a difference?

All of us are vulnerable to health care crises—our own and those of our families. At this time, the health care system is so complex that we are hard put to understand and deal with the problems of access to care and treatment when we are in these periods of vulnerability. Nurses understand the complexity of the health care environment and the consequences of unresolved and unaddressed health care issues.

Poll after poll tell us that the American public trusts nurses more than any other health professional or health institution. Of course, it is vital that any nurse candidate for public office or for a policy position must exemplify the reason for this trust. They must realize that their profession places them in a special place for the public's health. Their advocacy for patients and families must be viewed as central in all their work. Their care and concern for people must be translated into finding solutions to the pressing problems in health care today.

The issues we face in health care over the next few years will become more significant, not less. Increases in costs, cutbacks in services, and leaving out larger and larger numbers of people cannot be allowed to continue unchecked. Nurses have the guts, compassion, persistence, and vision to help solve these issues.

But what else do nurses bring to the table? Nurses have a bird's-eye view of our society and the influence of a broad array of health factors on the problems people face from birth to senescence. Nurses understand how health factors influence children's learning. Nurses understand how nutrition affects the way children face their day in school. Nurses understand the effects of sensory deprivation on youngsters and older people, and the needs that people have for environments that are not only loving—where possible—but enriched by activities which promote health. Do others have the depth of understanding that nurses have in these health and societal issues? Yes, for some, but not for others. Nurses have an unusually holistic approach to the way they view health and illness and the inter- action of social problems and health, an approach that is unex- celled by other clinicians. It is part of the way we think. The "public face" careers of the nurses described in this book give concrete examples of the way nurses think and put their knowl- edge to work in their public roles of advocacy for health and wel- fare. The thrilling stories in the book tell of the way nurses work and the way they bring their experiences and knowledge to bear on political issues. These stories illustrate nurses' abilities to organize, to build consensus, to "affect people's lives for the good," to focus on both the community and individuals as they promote public policy in health and related areas, as well as the most important social welfare issues facing our country today, such as Social Security.

Nurses bring knowledge, experience, and enormous commit- ment to political roles. They have the potential to be a strong voice for quality health care and the improvement of health serv- ices to all citizens across the spectrum of need.

So, given my assumption that nurses who run for public office or aim for high policy positions do exemplify the reasons for the public's trust, that they do realize that they hold a special place in advocating for patients and the public's health, that they are seeking solutions to the pressing problems in health care today—my unequivocal answer to my own questions has to be a resounding "yes."

This book tells the stories to back up my answer. But the book does more. It tells a wonderful story about nursing's beginnings and of the extraordinary accomplishments of the small group of women who helped to move mountains to develop the profession. Few can tell this story more effectively than it is told in the pages that follow. That story sets the stage for everything that current nurses have been able to accomplish. And against what odds did our pioneers work? And against what odds are our public policy careerists working today? The similarities and differences are shown clearly and with astonishing contemporary relevance. Some of the nurses talk about themselves as "breaking the mold." Others see their public policy lives as part of a continuum of nursing where they are putting their knowledge to work, as nurses, but in a more societal framework. However each individual nurse describes her career, the usefulness of these approaches, the specific lessons they offer, the humor, initiative, persistence, and drive they display are fascinating reading. But, more important, the background presented in this book and the wonderful stories it tells will inform, stimulate, and inspire current and future nurses. This book fills an important gap in nursing literature.

CLAIRE M. FAGIN, PhD, RN, FAAN

Introduction

We wrote this book to inspire nurses to seek public office and appointments. By illuminating the stories of nurses who have run for public office or who have been appointed to government positions, we hoped to inspire others to do likewise. We wanted nurses and other people interested in influencing health care policy and holding political office to have a book that they could refer to when engaging in political activism. The fact that there are nurses who hold such positions, having run successful campaigns, as well as those who have lost, often goes unnoticed by the majority of nurses and the public at large. Although still small in number, the fact that nurses hold political offices or political appointments challenges the historically held notion that nurses have had "little influence on the formulation of health care policy" (Leonard, 1994, p. 16). We wanted to put a face on these nurses so that they could be recognized and serve as role models for those to follow.

The idea for this book began with a conversation early in 1998 between Harriet Feldman and Dr. Ursula Springer, President of Springer Publishing Company. An interest in nurses who held office or were political appointees was initially kindled at the American Nurses Association convention that same year, where President Clinton spoke about the value nurses could bring to the political arena. It was Virginia Trotter Betts, then American Nurses Association President, who successfully brought the Association and the potential of nurses as a political body to the attention of the Clinton administration. As Harriet's thinking progressed, a number of questions kept coming up. For example, why did nurses pursue office or appointments, how did they go about it, and did people realize that they were nurses? It was time to put a face on these nurses who argued the case for better health care for the public. Hence, the title *Nurses in the Political Arena: The Public Face of Nursing* emerged. Since Sandy Lewenson's past research and interest concerned the political activity of nurses at the beginning of the 20th century, and she had experience as a book author, it was easy to persuade her to join in the writing of a book that would explore these and many other questions. Once our team was established, we began to formulate the ideas for the book. Following this, the publisher endorsed the project.

With the help of a graduate assistant, Lisette Barton, we spent many weeks collecting the names of nurses who held federal, state, and local positions, both elected and appointed. We did this by contacting the state nurses associations and the American Nurses Association as resources for names. We identified the *Directory of Capital Connection,* published by George Mason University, as a useful source of information. We also checked the archives of the Senate, and learned that there has never been a nurse who served as a United States Senator. During the interview held with Eddie Bernice Johnson, we learned that she was the first nurse to serve in the United States House of Representatives; she was elected to her first term in 1992. We sought the advice of nurse historians who were members of the American Association of the History of Nurses. Through this resource, we were able to uncover the name of one nurse who ran for office in 1920, Margaret Brydon Laird, following the passage of women suffrage, and a second nurse, Eloise Nagel, who was elected in 1972 as mayor of Shrewsbury Township in New Jersey. Coincidentally, while interviewing Imogene King for the Centennial Celebration of Teachers College, Columbia University, we learned that she had been elected alderman of Wood Dale, Illinois in 1975.

As the weeks progressed, we developed a method for identifying and cataloging the names of nurses who had run for public office as well as those nurses who held appointed governmental positions. We claim to have neither a complete list nor one that is exhaustive. Still, we believe that our list of more than 120 nurses in public service represents the majority of the nurses who hold public office and a representative number of those who have been appointed. Those nurses who ran for office and lost were harder to find since they aren't found in congressional records or organizational listings. A number of additional names came from word of mouth from those people we interviewed and others that had heard about the book.

In preparing a list of nurses to be interviewed, we wanted to have a broad spectrum of types of positions held as well as representation from different geographical areas throughout the United States. We received funding through a Pace University Kenan Research grant to purchase two tape recorders and subsidize some of the interview transcriptions. We conducted the interviews between January 1999 and November 1999. At the same time, we reviewed current and past articles and books that focused on political activism and nursing. We decided that while we would engage in a rigorous interview process, this would not be a phenomenological study. Nor do we consider it a historical research study. Yet, as with qualitative research, we methodically examined the data for themes that emerged and stories that could be told. Direct quotes appear with permission and participants' names and affiliations appear in the Appendix.

Most heartening for us was the response we received during the interviews. Many of the nurses we interviewed cheered us on, saying things such as, "It's about time something like this was published," "What a great idea," "I could have used this book when I ran for office!" and "A book like yours will help people get to the table . . . nurses need to stretch themselves." Those nurses immediately recognized the relevance of the book to the work they were doing. They also noted that the book would encourage others in nursing who might never have known about or thought to follow a similar path. While collecting the interviews, we began the process of writing. How to tell the stories and fit them into a coherent whole required a great deal of discussion, as well as many sessions of writing, editing, and rewriting. We wanted readers to share in the stories of the nurses themselves; so wherever we could do so, we used their own words.

In addition to the many common themes that emerged, we learned that this group of nurses was not of one mind or political bent. They brought their own ideas about political issues and their own stories about how and why they got where they were. We recognized, too, that there were almost as many different approaches or responses to political solutions as there were similarities. For example, we had thought that overwhelmingly nurses would support pro-choice, and were surprised when more than a few supported pro-life. Our gut feeling that nearly all nurses were Democratic was challenged by the fact that while about 60% were Democrats, 25% were Republicans and the remainder were identified as Independent or undeclared. Some of those individuals who were appointed to positions rather than elected stated that they had to maintain a bipartisan stance rather than having allegiance to a single party, and so they declared no affiliation.

Chapter 1, *Nurses in the Political Process: The Face That No One Sees,* provides an overview of the book. Initially, there is a discussion of the lack of recognition of the political activities of nurses and the reason that nurses are needed at the table. The stages of political development are used as a backdrop for understanding the political activism of the nurses interviewed. The chapter presents the questions raised during the interviews, as well as the major themes we discovered. We tried to identify each of the nurses we interviewed, introducing them to the reader by way of these themes.

In chapter 2, *Historical Perspective on Nurses Active in the Political Process,* we explore the historical nature of nurses and nursing, including political activity at the beginning of the 20th century and how nurses influenced the political issues of the day. We introduce a brief description of how nursing schools began and how the professional organizations formed. Nursing organizations, considered by the first editor of the *American Journal of Nursing,* Sophia Palmer, to be the "power of the day" (Palmer, 1991, p. 297), served as the political vehicle for nurses trying to establish educational and practice standards. We also discuss the meaning of *nursism,* a term used to describe how nurses have experienced prejudice toward the caring role (Lewenson, 1996). We look at the effect of the woman's movement of the beginning of the century, and during the 1960s and 1970s, on the nursing profession and nurses. The connection with our history is also demonstrated at the opening of each chapter, where we use what we believe to be significant historical quotes.

In chapter 3, *Nurses in the Political Arena: The Face the Public Sees* we provide a demographic summary of the nurses interviewed. This chapter is divided into sections describing the nurse who holds a public position; how opportunities to serve were created; the passion connected with their service; how political skills were developed; the effective use of power; the need to have breadth of knowledge; and how grassroots activism is used to connect with people and "get the job done." We uncover the tragedies and untoward experiences that led some of the nurses to run for office or seek political appointments and, alternately, the impetus provided by their desire to improve the ills of society. The period of social and political change marked by the '60s and '70s provided the drive in some for participation in public service.

Chapter 4, *Nurses' Action on Social Issues* examines the nurse as a social force in history and the present, and looks at the major issues nurses have brought to the table. These issues include using gains of tobacco control initiatives, addressing mental health, supporting seniors, advocating healthy children, championing women's issues, responding to the HIV/AIDS epidemic, advancing nursing practice, shaping insurance reform, leading health care reform, and tackling other pressing social issues. In this chapter we also use the stories of the nurses interviewed to describe their impact on political processes and outcomes.

In chapter 5, *Negotiating the Political Process: Lessons Learned* we explore the lessons learned by the candidates and the elected and appointed nurses. This chapter discusses 11 lessons that the nurses who were interviewed shared with us. For example, "It takes a personal investment of time, money, and energy," illustrates the tremendous energy required to run for public office. Standing out in the cold at dawn, or spending weekends at endless fundraiser events, are part of the daily experiences of those who ran for office. Another lesson is the need to develop a thick skin. Politics can be rough, and nurses need to be ready to negotiate in such a setting. Yet another lesson is how difficult it is to fundraise, particularly knowing how important it was to their success.

In chapter 6, *Creating Political Opportunities,* we provide insights on winning, dealing with defeat, and how to get elected or appointed, as well as general advice shared by the nurses interviewed. Their advice includes such things as reading the paper daily, getting involved in a political party, presenting the "right" image, knowing your community, starting local, learning to fundraise, having a sense of humor, and knowing that family support is essential. Also addressed is the public trust that nurses enjoy and ways that nurses have created political opportunities in order to accomplish their personal and professional goals.

In addition to the six chapters, we include appendices identifying each person interviewed, his or her title, and date of interview and a list of political action databases and audiovisuals on nurses and politics. Along with this, we include a sample of some of the items used in the campaigns of those who ran for public office (Appendix C). Whether they won or lost, each of the individuals who engaged in this political activity gave it their fullest attention and should be recognized for doing so. Their stories, told within the chapters of this book, will hopefully inspire others to move in a similar direction. Nurses are concerned about their communities and about people living in those communities. Without their care and expertise, many of the necessary primary health care services that citizens receive would be lost. In the tradition of the late 19th and early 20th century public health nurses, the elected and appointed nurses of today, as well as the nurses who are politically active individually and through professional organizations, clearly recognize the relationship between the health of their constituents and their political obligation to advocate change.

The writing of this book has been both a pleasure and a learning experience. We spent blocks of time together planning, developing the themes, and creating many opportunities to discuss our values and our dreams about nursing's future. Our goal in completing this book was to put a "face" on the people we interviewed. The process of writing required each of us to understand our own background and ideas about political activism. Also, our own stories emerged as we read and interpreted the stories of those interviewed. This created a dynamic exchange that continued during the process of writing.

We hope to use this book, as others might, in undergraduate and graduate nursing classrooms. Further, the book can serve as an impetus for dialogue about our nursing leaders, nurses who hold political office, those who risked the election process, and those who shape public policy daily in their positions as government appointees. Nurses in clinical practice and nurses who wish to enrich their knowledge of political action would also benefit from this work. This book may be of relevance as well to special interest groups that have an area of expertise that could be used to help shape public policy.

The people we interviewed all expressed an interest in this publication. Many expressed their feelings that it could help bring others along and indicated that they wished they had had such a guide when they started their own journey into politics. They saw the value this work will have for future generations and felt encouraged by it. They saw themselves as part of a larger political picture where they could make changes in policy that would benefit society—some working behind the scenes where they could make the most impact and change, and others as politicians.

In summary, we hope this book will motivate other nurses to take risks and seek public office or political appointment, just as the risk takers did during the times of Lillian Wald, Lavinia Dock, and Margaret Sanger. It took until 1992, 78 years after the passage of women's suffrage, before a nurse entered the United States House of Representatives. As of 2000, we still do not have a nurse in the Senate. The time has clearly come. In fact, one of the individuals discussed in the book, The Honorable Janegale Boyd of the Florida House of Representatives, announced at the time of this writing that she is running for the United State Senate as a candidate from Florida. Although Representative Boyd was not available for interview, her comments were taken from a presentation heard by Harriet at the November 1999 meeting of the American Academy of Nursing. Boyd's win would be a first for nurses. We cannot let another year go by before we enter the Senate. Nurses have the knowledge and skills; we just need to show our "face."

HARRIET R. FELDMAN, PhD, RN, FAAN
SANDRA B. LEWENSON, EdD, RN

REFERENCES

Leonard, M. (1994). Levels of political participation and political expectations among nurses in New York State. *Journal of the New York State Nurses Association, 25*(1), 16–20.

Lewenson, S. B. (1996). *Taking charge: Nursing, suffrage, and feminism in America, 1873–1920.* New York: National League for Nursing Press.

Palmer, S. (1991). Training school alumnae associations. In N. Brinbach & S. B. Lewenson (Eds.), *First words: Selected addresses from the National League for Nursing, 1894–1933* (pp. 293–297). New York: National League for Nursing Press. (Original work published in 1897).

CHAPTER ONE

Nurses in the Political Process: The Face That No One Sees

Government shapes literally every aspect of our lives in some form or another. The real question is whether we passively allow ourselves to be impacted by government or whether we attempt to impact government ourselves, to attempt to beneficially shape the outcomes.

—Federici

WHY ARE NURSES NEEDED AT THE TABLE?

Nurses care. They roll up their sleeves and do their work. Nurses are out there on the front line, listening to families, knocking on doors, working in schools, and being involved with the lives of people living in the community. Nurses are accustomed to "dirty business." A nurse changes dressings, carries bedpans, and deals with the most intimate parts of human life. Politics is dirty business, too. Politicians also roll up their sleeves and argue, debate, and proverbially "change bedpans" in order to change the social order. Politicians involve themselves in the lives of their constituents. They want to improve the day-to-day lives of people and do so by changing the laws and policies that govern. Firmly grounded in the concepts of primary health care, nurses change the lives of individuals, families, and communities by knowing what needs to be changed and then doing the "hands-on" business.

Although nurses deal with many of the same topics addressed by local, state, and federal government, they often bury themselves in minutiae. For example, they may spend an inordinate amount of time with one patient or one small unit, or spend hours obtaining Medicaid coverage for one person. As a result, they may lose sight of the "bigger picture." Sometimes they haven't even given thought to the fact that there is a "bigger picture." But because their education and experience give them the knowledge and skills to make change, nurses can take an active role in the everyday lives of people, and they can learn the work of public service. Backer, Costello-Nikitas, Mason, McBride, and Vance (1993) are in agreement with this position, saying, "Nurses and other women have the potential to transform public policies. Such transformation can instill an ethic of caring into health policies that value and promote the health and wholeness of individuals, families, and communities" (p. 69).

Few people are likely to know nurses who serve in the public arena. For most nurses, political activism is an abstract term, or at best involves writing a letter to one's representative or volunteering to work on a local campaign. Nursing organizations invest more directly in the political process by supporting political action, mainly through contributions and lobbying. They have established political action groups, for example, state and federal political action committees and N-STAT (Nurses Strategic Action Team), an American Nurses Association grassroots lobbying group comprised of individual state nurses association members. Although there is great potential for these organizations to be effective, membership has fallen in many of the state nurses associations, and too often nurses do not recognize their strength or potential contributions beyond the clinical practice arena. As well, there may be many reasons that keep nurses from recognizing their abilities. One explanation is *nursism,* the term that describes the prejudice that nurses experience in their professional lives (Lewenson, 1996). Although nurses are trusted, as so many of the people interviewed said, they are not always valued. Nurses have been relegated to a lower socioeconomic status than other professions. "How the educated young women may be interested in this work of ours which is paradoxical in offering so much and so little—so much opportunity for usefulness and so little worldly advancement" (Riddle, 1911/1993, p. 84).

When interviewed for this book, United States Representative Lois Capps said:

> If we could harness the political energy of every nurse in this country, look what we could do . . . We could change the business

in the direction we need to go . . . to be more humane, more caring, more just, more protective of young children and older people.

The more than 2,500,000 nurses in the United States can generate a formidable amount of political energy to "beneficially shape the outcomes" (Federici, 1996, p. 16).

Mason, Backer, and Georges (1991) make two assumptions in their discussion of a feminist model of empowerment: that "nurses collectively and individually have more potential than currently is manifest, and that increasing nurses' political awareness and skills is necessary to bring about changes in a troubled health care system" (p. 72). These assumptions were borne out in our interviews with elected and appointed officials. Among the reasons they cited for nurses to be at the table were their strong overriding belief in public service and strong sense of community, their advocacy role, their commitment to access to health care, their ability to work with people where they are on their terms, their "grassroots" skills, and the high degree of trust that nurses have from others. Nurses need to debate the key issues that promote the public's interests and needs. As a social force, they also must be part of the solutions to problems and concerns, acting for "collectivism, cooperation, and equality" (Gil, 1981). Building on the important skills nurses possess—for example, listening, observing, communicating, leading, negotiating, and a unique perspective on human life—and learning the systems and structures of attaining and being successful in one's public position, nurses have been able to make a difference.

While the nursing literature of the 1980s attested to the potential of nurses, also featured was their perceived powerlessness to shape the outcomes of health care and even their own clinical practice (Bullough & Bullough, 1984; Ferguson, 1985; Hayes & Fritsch, 1988; Maraldo, 1985). Although individual nurses held high-level appointments and offices at that time, overall, there were few political role models, and the internal struggles within nursing itself diverted organized nursing from becoming politically relevant and from fulfilling its potential to influence important health and social issues. Hayes and Fritsch (1988) wrote: "Nurses, should they remain ignorant politically, will not have a voice in the allocation of resources they say their clients must have" (p. 33).

During this pivotal time in nursing's history, there was also a call to arms to become visible, develop political skills, learn how to use power, and become advocates for health care consumers on a much broader scale (Lerner, 1985; Schutzenhofer & Cannon, 1986). Prior to the realization that, given the development of political awareness and skills, nurses had an important role to play in advancing public and health policy, nurses had been largely invisible at the political table. This was characteristic of the culture of nursing of the past, which highly valued selfless and self-effacing behavior and advanced the supportive (handmaiden) rather than the leadership role of nurses—the person in the background, the "face that no one sees." Only recently has the literature reflected nursing's political activism at the beginning of the 20th century. Nursing's political activism, however, remains virtually "faceless" and still needs to be uncovered.

THE FOUR STAGES OF NURSING'S POLITICAL DEVELOPMENT

Cohen et al. (1996), in an effort to "systematically analyze the evolution of nursing as a body politic" (p. 259), developed a framework for understanding nursing's involvement in the political arena. The four stages are: "Buy-in," "Self-interest," "Political sophistication," and "Leading the way."

The first stage highlights the awareness and importance of political activism for attaining professional goals. Issues of power and a recognition that nurses need to be involved in politics to have input in health care policy decision-making mark the essence of this stage. The second, or self-interest, stage, perhaps most prevalent in the late 1970s and early 1980s, involves activities that identify the profession within the political arena. This is where political activism enhances and promotes nursing's self-interest, which Stevens (1985) refers to as "nursing's own internal, intraprofessional concerns" (p. 17). MacPherson (1987) sees this view in a less flattering light, saying that "Instead of looking at structural problems in the health care system that will require long-term sweeping changes, nursing leaders, on the whole, tend to concentrate on enhancing the power of nursing" (p. 9). Kate Malliarakis, Branch Chief of Specific Drugs of the Office of National

Drug Control Policy calls this the "myopia of nursing." It is important to note, however, that in this second stage coalitions are built creating a strong political base for future activism. Stage three, political sophistication, is the result of complex political activity and an already established political foothold in government. Exemplars of this stage include the appointment of nurses to federal positions, where nursing expertise is acknowledged and sought, and the election of nurses to public office.

The final stage is where nursing leaders are appointed to important governmental positions and elected leaders set the course for change. According to Terry (1993), "political leadership does not adapt to change but initiates change, focusing either on accomplishing the will of the leader (power over) or the will of the followers (power with)" (p. 31). Those who reach the stage of leading the way "become initiators of crucial health policy ideas and innovations as instigators, leaders, or formulators of health policy" (Cohen et al., 1996, p. 263). For example, while serving as a Congressional Science Fellow in the Office of Senator Daniel K. Inouye (D-Hawaii), Lescavage (1995) focused on "participating in the resolution of national health care reform, becoming an authority on the legislative process and its application to health care, and working as a congressional staffer on the Defense Appropriations Subcommittee" (p. 18). She believes that the presence of nurses in Washington "and beyond" is being felt more than ever. The fact that nurses were on the task force that addressed health care reform in the 1990s led her to say "The Clintons' affirmation of our profession is obvious. Indeed this type of Presidential recognition is a first" (p. 20).

Cohen et al. (1996) state that the four stages are not time-bound; that no stage is more important than another; and that nursing often straddles the different stages depending on the issues at hand. As well, individual nurses may find themselves at different levels, depending on the level of their political involvement and their political sophistication. Cindy Empson, Kansas State Legislator, believes that, "Nurses are unique in compassion and the belief that they can help people. They are special individuals who should be in political office." While scores of articles have been written on political action by nurses, as well as serving in supportive and even influential roles, few have been published on the leadership role of nurses in appointed and elected public positions.

PUTTING ON A FACE

Of the 435 members of the United States House of Representatives, three in the 106th Congress (1999) were nurses: Representative Lois Capps, RN (D-California), Representative Eddie Bernice Johnson, RN (D-Texas), and Carolyn McCarthy, LPN (D-New York). Approximately 70 nurses were identified as representatives in their state legislatures. During 1998–1999, a number of nurses held key appointed positions in the state and federal governments, for example, Deputy Commissioner of Health and Senior Services in New Jersey, Senior Program and Policy Specialist in the United States Office of Special Education, Director of the Occupational Safety and Health Administration (OSHA), Trial Attorney in the United States Department of Justice, Senior Advisor on Nursing and Policy to the Secretary and Assistant Secretary of Health, United States Department of Health and Human Services (DHHS), Borough President of Queens, New York, and Special Assistant to the Under Secretary for Health, United States Department of Veteran Affairs.

The elected and appointed officials presented throughout this book are individuals who have visibly affected government and, consequently, beneficially shaped the policies, practices, and laws that affect the health and welfare of the citizens of the United States. Although many may still argue that nurses are not at the "table" in the public arena, and, indeed, a small minority of those interviewed for this book would agree, conversations with the majority of those interviewed have begun to tell a very different story.

To gather information about nurses in public positions, more than 45 nurses were interviewed over the course of about 10 months. They were asked to share their perspectives on their current and past positions in public service, using the following prompts.

- Tell me about your background in nursing and what led you to this position.
- How did your background in nursing influence the decisions you made?
- Do you tell others about your nursing background?
- Do people see you differently because you are a nurse?

- What issues have you brought or helped others to bring to the table?
- What impact have you made on political processes and outcomes?
- How did you develop the political skills needed to carry out your work?
- Why did you get involved in public service?
- How do you interface with the public?
- Was there anyone who served as a mentor in guiding you or getting you into your past/present position?
- Were you elected or appointed, and what was the process involved in the election/appointment?
- How did your political party affiliation contribute to your election/appointment?
- How did you find financial backing for your candidacy (if elected)?
- What advice would you give to others who may be interested in an appointment or public office?

Further questions that arose based on their responses were asked to get a better understanding of the role and background of the individuals who were interviewed. In fact, some of these questions were asked of subsequent participants. In the case of those who ran for office and were not elected, questions were refocused to fit their situation. For example, they were asked, "What issues did your campaign focus on?" "What was the most important thing you learned from the experience of running for office?" "What role did political party affiliation play in the campaign process, including losing the election?" and "Would you consider running or do you plan to run again?" The interviews were conducted by telephone and were tape-recorded, with permission. We also took copious notes of our conversations, reviewed each other's notes and audiotapes, and held many work sessions to discuss the interviews, develop profiles and demographic summaries, identify themes, and come to a sense of the impact on health and public policy being made by nurses.

Over and over again, we were struck by the recurring themes. The themes presented themselves as: public trust and credibility, advocacy, breadth of knowledge and influence, using expertise and background to advance the agenda, being part of the solution,

making a difference, putting a "face" on the policy, using the nursing process to guide one's thinking, getting to the table, grassroots
involvement and community service, being a health resource,
nursing skills as political skills, having "fire in the belly" (being
passionate about what you do), having previous exposure to
political behavior, the presence of mentors and role models, caring on a "grand scale," and pioneering efforts of these nurses.
The numerous anecdotes that follow on the next several pages
put a face on these themes and provide a context for the chapters that follow.

PUBLIC TRUST AND CREDIBILITY

"Nurses have credibility and respect. People trust us, and they
should" (Capps, 1998, p. 80). Not only does the public hold nurses
in high regard, politicians recognize this, and actively seek their
opinions. In describing her campaign strategizing, Robson (1998)
said that nurses have "an intrinsically positive image. Nurses
project a natural image of trustworthiness, honesty, and caring,
qualities not often associated with politicians. This message
sparked interest and ignited the campaign" (p. 428). When interviewed, Representative Lois Capps said that nurses know they
are trusted. It is not uncommon to hear that nurses are seen as
the most trusted of professionals. Christine E. Canavan, Massachusetts State Legislator, says that "Nurses are held in high
esteem. People contact you because they have a problem. Nurses
solve problems!" Patricia Montoya, Commissioner for Children,
Youth, and Families for the United States Department of Health
and Human Services, said that nurses don't understand what
their impact is on people; "Nurses are highly respected and
trusted." She found that when lobbying, legislators saw her as a
lobbyist but trusted her as someone who would "tell the truth."
She said that we should be using this trust to our advantage to
advance the profession.

On her walk through the entire city she would later represent
as a Massachusetts State Legislator, Mary Jane Simmons built
credibility by asking constituents what they perceived as assets
and what they thought needed improvement. People would comment that no one ever asked them what they wanted to see
changed. She also didn't make any promises, but instead shared

her vision and some of the major things she wanted to do if elected. Once elected she said, "My best ideas come from my constituents. [I tell them] 'let me know because I can't think of everything.'" Connecticut State Legislator Mary McGrattan said that in her last campaign the fact that she was a registered nurse gave some credibility to her position on managed care. People could "associate that I'm a nurse, that I know and I understand."

ADVOCACY

Nurses advocate; political leaders need to advocate. Nurses who either hold office or are national or state appointees have the opportunity to advocate for large groups of people and communities, and to make changes in policies and laws. The ability to convince others while serving in a public position is essential for real change. Allison Giles, formerly an aide to Congressman Bill Thomas (R-California) and Professional Staff of the Health Subcommittee of the House Ways and Means Committee, spoke about being seen as a patient advocate. She said that her experience with patients and families helped her "see some of the holes in the system, areas that could be improved to create better patient outcomes." She viewed patient advocacy as the part of her background most useful in her public role, that is, knowing

> The frustration that patients and families may feel when they're in a hospital or in a setting where decisions are made that are beyond their control or are very confusing, whether they are dealing with insurance companies, dealing with hospital administrators, dealing with physicians, trying to translate some of the complicated issues to "how does this affect me, my health."

Lois Capps sees herself as an advocate for her constituents. In deciding to run for office to take the seat of her husband, who had died following a car accident, she was struck that the two issues high on her priority list—health care and education—were of great importance in her district and ones she knew well. Being a school nurse provided her with the depth and understanding she needed to address these issues, as well as a way for her to continue her strong advocacy for children and families. Motivated by the death of her secretary, Georgia State Representative Sharon Cooper advocated for a shorter waiting period for the approval of experimental drugs. Advocating health care for employees of the Federal Aviation Administration (FAA), Irma Hart inaugurated and is now National Manager of the Health Awareness Program that gained national status in 1990. She also has been an advocate for nurses, increasing the number within the FAA, raising the grade of nurses hired for the program, and developing a manual that nurses could use to educate clients. As an advocate for citizens in the 10 counties she serves, Florida State Representative Janegale Boyd sponsored a due process bill. This bill allows patients to stay with their provider/s even if their health insurance company drops them, by extending the time period of coverage by 6 months.

BREADTH OF KNOWLEDGE AND EXPERIENCE

The application of nursing knowledge and experience to public service illustrates an expanded definition of nursing. What we value in our nursing background, for example, education, practice, and research, as well as the skills garnered in earning the title of nurse, enables nurses to practice in alternative arenas. The traditional myth of the typical "hospital" role of the nurse is being challenged daily by nurses who practice their profession in the public sector. Holding public office, running for office, or being appointed to public service provide outstanding opportunities to practice what has been learned in nursing. Philadelphia Deputy Commissioner of Health Donna Gentile O'Donnell aptly said, "If you can organize a patient ward, you can organize a political ward." Moving into a nontraditional role in informatics created an opportunity for Lieutenant Colonel Rosemary Nelson to demonstrate her expertise in technology for health care delivery. She was instrumental in developing a computerized patient record, worldwide, for the Department of Defense. This is a longitudinal record that moves with the patient, both active military and their families and veterans. Through her know-how and performance, she "broke the mold regarding the general opinion of nurses by others." It was the value of her nursing background and its service orientation that brought Shirley Chater, former Commissioner of the United States Social Security Administration, to her federal appointment. Chater used the skills she learned in her nursing curriculum, e.g., people skills, communication, listening, observation, and empathy, to make the Social Security Administration more customer-focused.

USING EXPERTISE AND BACKGROUND TO ADVANCE THE AGENDA

The nurses who ran for public office, who currently hold or have held office, or who were appointed to leadership positions in government attributed much of their success to their nursing background. When they told their stories, they acknowledged that something in their nursing backgrounds—whether it was education, practice, research, or professional connections—had contributed to their ability to serve the public. These nurses demonstrate a unique application of their profession to a much larger setting than nurses typically work in. For example, Claire Shulman, Borough President of Queens in New York City, noted that she was caring for the whole borough when she cited the high number of recent immigrants in her constituency and her efforts to begin a borough-wide immunization program. While telling her story, she recognized that her nursing practice continued in her political position, much as it did in her earlier years in the hospital, but she was now applying nursing principles and ideas to addressing the larger social, political, and economic issues that she found in her community of Queens, New York. Her agenda included the delivery of medical services, immunization for children, and the delivery of primary care to the citizens of Queens.

Marilyn Goldwater, Maryland State Legislator and Deputy Majority Leader, is seen as an expert on health issues. Because of her expertise she was able to pull together people from the nursing community to advance legislation in the 1970s and 1980s to reimburse nurse midwives and nurse anesthetists. Reporters came to her for her knowledge of health care, as did colleagues in the legislature. She took the lead on legislation to enact changes in health maintenance organizations (HMOs), including the requirement that they offer point-of-service plans, have access to obstetric and gynecologic services, and abolish "drive-through" delivery and mastectomy. Because of her nursing background, Herschella Horton, Arizona State Legislator, says she is a voice of reality in the political process. She educates others and is persuasive in health care matters, especially behavioral health. She tries to teach people how to be effective, for example, how to impact the political process and make your voice heard.

BEING PART OF THE SOLUTION

When asked to give advice to others, Eve Franklin, Montana State Legislator said, "If you care about the world, it is power. You affect people's lives for the good. Being an 'insider' is critical." As someone who was clearly "part of the solution," she worked toward creating positive change in health care in the state while she was in office. She said that if nurses were not there every step of the way, "There would not be reimbursement for advanced practice nurses in Montana." She also commented that the language of bills is important, and that nurses can influence this through their involvement in the political process. Carolyn McCarthy became involved in the political process after being challenged by a reporter who asked if she was "mad enough to run" following an attempt to repeal the ban on assault weapons. Her husband and son had been shot on a commuter train in a random act of violence. She was outraged when her own congressman voted in favor of repeal. She said this of her impact on political processes:

> I think the biggest effect I've had on legislation is that I am able to work with both parties to find consensus that will move legislation forward. In addition, I think I have been able to remind a lot of members that people back home listen and if they don't like what they hear, they might find themselves running against an upset nurse/housewife.

In her role as Chief of Staff to Senator Quentin Burdick (D-North Dakota), Mary Wakefield drafted many health-related initiatives, "analyzing the impact of legislation on health, and handling a variety of constituent concerns related to these issues . . . [This enabled her to] take my healthcare background and education and bring it to bear on public policy" ("An interview with Mary Wakefield," 1992, p. 14). In late 1999, Wakefield was appointed to a 3-year term as a commissioner to the Medicare Payment Advisory Commission (MedPAC), a 15-member nonpartisan group that "advises Congress on Medicare payment policies through research, reports, and recommendations. This is her second appointment to a health care commission—she previously served on the President's Advisory Commission on Consumer Protection and Quality in the Health Care Industry" (SNA members appointed, 1999). When she moved into her condominium in suburban Chicago, Imogene King thought it important to get involved in her community. At the time, she observed that children were in potential danger playing in a "deep hole that was dug for a foundation." She tried to organize other residents and suggested that they go to city hall. She was elected president of the condominium and went to city hall alone. She proposed a "simple solution of moving dirt from one building site to the hole." Through the process of solving this problem she became to known to the mayor, who encouraged her to run for alderman in her community.

MAKING A DIFFERENCE

During her nursing education, Virginia Trotter Betts, Senior Advisor on Nursing and Policy to the Secretary and Assistant Secretary of Health, DHHS, was asked by her faculty to "make a difference in the lives of people." She has used her past positions, including President of the American Nurses Association, and her present position to make a difference with larger groups through public policy. As Senior Advisor on Nursing and Policy, she has tried to focus on a provider- vs. physician-based model, so that wherever "physician" is mentioned in legislation or policy the term "provider" would be used to enable nurses and other health care providers to have a place at the table. As former Chief of Staff to Senator Robert Dole (R-Kansas), Sheila Burke felt that she made a difference in terms of how issues were drafted, including Medicare and Medicaid legislation, nurse practitioner reimbursement, financing rural clinics, and coverage for hospice and home care within the Medicare program. DeParle (1995) said this of Sheila Burke: "Burke is sometimes called 'the 101st Senator,' a title that, for all its hyperbole, technically understates her role. Day to day, Burke does more to shape the Senate's agenda than all but a handful of its actual members" (p. 34).

Bonnie Ryan, Chief, Veterans Administration Home and Community-Based Care, has her roots in community nursing and hospice care. While serving on the board of a state hospice organization in Illinois, she was successful in a grassroots effort to lobby for state Medicaid restoration of benefits for hospice. She brought together diverse people in the hospice community around a common purpose/cause to make a difference. She also was involved in a three-state public advocacy committee to work on end-of-life legislation. Later, she organized a national summit on end-of-life care. Muriel Shore, Mayor of Fairfield, New Jersey, has made a difference in the lives of seniors through several quality-of-life initiatives, for example, creation of a Senior Resource Center where seniors can learn technology, and LIFES, a program for seniors that focuses on health and activities of daily living. She feels strongly that "nurses can make a difference" by focusing on community, getting involved in health care issues, and volunteering.

PUTTING A "FACE" ON THE POLICY

Pennsylvania State Representative Patricia Vance was able to successfully advance legislation under the Pennsylvania Drug and Alcohol Law in changing the age at which a child was considered an adult from 14 to 18. More than once, the bill had been stalled in the Senate. When interviewed, Representative Vance spoke about a woman who knew her son was on drugs and was in "desperate trouble," but was helpless to intervene because he was legally designated as an adult. "Primarily we got it [the legislation] passed through the Senate because this woman's son committed suicide in their family room." That tragedy put a "face" on the bill. Former Rhode Island State Senator Joseph Polisena said that by being a nurse he had a perspective that others didn't have. In 6 years, "I had over 30 bills become law . . . most of them were health bills." He would say to the other legislators, "Think of your mother, think of your father, think of your children, think of your wife. I'd hold the bill up and put a face on it, trying to get to their emotions." He would also challenge other legislators and lobbyists when health issues came up and were being misrepresented. He could clear up the misconceptions and properly represent the policy or issue.

Eileen Cody, Washington State Legislator, relayed a story about how she influenced the Washington State House of Representatives to pass legislation to support breastfeeding in the workplace. The House vote came about in a session where Representative Cody filled the gallery with women who sat there and breastfed their babies. Although the Senate defeated the bill, it was to be reintroduced the following year, beginning again with the House. When she told a colleague in the Washington House of Representatives that she intended to reintroduce the bill, he responded, "You're not going to bring in those women again, are you?"

Using the Nursing Process to Guide One's Thinking

Many of those interviewed talked about how the nursing process framed their thinking about problems and issues and gave them the ability to come up with solutions. This knowledge was easily transferred from their nursing background to their life in politics and policy. The process of assessment, planning, implementation, and evaluation can be applied to organizational change, team-building, research, strategic planning, and so many other activities. As liaison to the White House for Women's Affairs, Nancy Valentine wrote a proposal for a national Stop Smoking campaign. She conducted a literature search, talked to people, and knew how to access information. These typical nursing process skills were used frequently in problem solving and research. Beth Mazzella, Chief Nurse of the United States Public Health Service, in describing how her nursing background influenced the decisions made, referred to two ingredients: the nursing process and caring. She said that the nursing process is used to guide critical thinking and "that it is something that you do automatically . . . you sit down and take stock . . . what are the needs, what are the causes of the problem, how do we intervene, were we successful, and why or why not?" Mary Eileen (Mel) Callan, Nurse Practitioner in Rochester and former candidate for state and county positions in New York, said that she used the nursing process to develop her campaign strategy.

A final illustration attests to the use of the nursing process to guide one's thinking in the political arena. As reported in an article that appeared in *Nursing Administration Quarterly,* Virginia Trotter Betts (1996) described her involvement in the health care reform debate through a Task Force spearheaded by the American Nurses Association. She said that the first step of the Task Force was to "get our arms around 'the health care crisis,' to accurately name the problem(s) in health care before we began delineating solutions" (p. 1). She went on to elaborate the importance of assessment and further said that "without a full and accurate diagnosis, governmental solutions have only a happenstance of 'curing' their ill-defined problems" (p. 1). So, despite the negative press the nursing process often gets, its value was immeasurable for so many of the people who were interviewed.

GETTING TO THE TABLE

Some nurses share the perspective of Mary Wakefield that "it is very appropriate for nursing to be wherever the table may be"; others questioned whether or not nurses are even "at the table." For example, Kate Malliarakis, Branch Chief of Specific Drugs for the Office of National Drug Control Policy, said, "We are not even at the table . . . we are not there politically nor professionally." She was emphatic in saying, however, that nurses need to fight to get to the table. We belong there. Virginia Trotter Betts has had progressively more to say at the table, having gotten her start as a health legislative assistant to then-Senator Albert Gore, and now as Senior Advisor on Nursing and Policy in the Department of Health and Human Services (DHHS). Although she has helped to raise the presence of nursing in DHHS, she said, "We have miles to go . . . the job of leaders is to tell the nursing story." Newer to the federal scene is Beverly Malone, who was appointed in January 2000 to the position of Deputy Assistant Secretary for Health within the DHHS. In a press release about her appointment, Malone said, "I look forward to bringing nursing's perspective to the table at this important policy-setting level" (Beverly Malone Appointed to Key Federal Position, 1999, p. 2).

When she chaired the committee to revise the Nurse Practice Act in New Jersey in the early 1970s, New Jersey Assemblywoman Barbara Wright learned a lot about being at the table. The new definition of nursing included language about physical and emotional health. According to Wright, the inclusion of emotional health was accomplished because "a Rutgers [University]-educated psych nurse was sitting at the table. If you think being at the table makes a difference, believe me it did. We had many debates. They were often focused on those two important words." Patricia Montoya got to the table by working on a friend's political campaign. His optimism and vision were inspiring and she learned that when you "support the issues of others you can move your own issues forward." Because she supported the issues of a New Mexico legislator, she was able to move ahead the nurse practice act in that state. She and her nursing friends helped educate him and he, in turn, brought her ideas to the table. This experience got her "hooked" on politics. Further, legislators working on health issues welcomed her expertise.

GRASSROOTS INVOLVEMENT AND COMMUNITY SERVICE

The environment in which many of these nurses matured as professionals fostered the feeling of community service. Kay Khan, a 1965 graduate of Boston University, began giving back to the country by joining the Peace Corps. She has continued to serve the public in her role as Massachusetts State Legislator, noting that public policy and nursing go hand in hand. For some of the nurses, their participation in community service was a carry-over from their experiences growing up in their families of origin. Likewise, Oregon State Representative Judy Uherbelau joined the Peace Corps. She said that she always felt you had to "give back something to the community." Mary Jane Simmons described herself as coming from a political family. Her father was a politician and her mother was a nurse. Simmons entered public service because of her concern with community issues, such as overcrowding and sewage problems. Her mother had always encouraged volunteerism and told her she could do anything she wanted to do. Entry into political life was just another way to help people. Pat Latona's involvement in her community led her to seek a position on the town board in Mamaroneck, New York. For example, she had been Traffic Commissioner and Deputy Chairperson of her planning board. Many of those interviewed expressed a desire to serve their communities, to use what they had learned to make changes they knew to be important and relevant to health care. They had a strong sense of a commitment to community and wanted to "give back." Many became involved in local parent-teachers associations when their children were small. Others became involved because of a local political issue that affected their home or family.

Overwhelmingly, their common history of volunteerism was evident. Nancy McKelvey, Chief Nurse of the American Red Cross, spoke of her lifelong background as a volunteer in her community and church. She pointed out, however, that altruism was not enough; "You must have the skills to influence change." To convert one's sense of community and good citizenship requires the development of the political skills needed to create a healthier society. She has long had a commitment to "giving back." Marilyn Lee, Hawaii State Representative, spoke of her earliest public service as a Girl Scout who assisted poor people in the community, to her role as a Foreign Service wife, her involvement as president of her local parent-teacher association, and her service as a member of her community advisory board. In describing her family, New York Assemblywoman Maureen O'Connell said, "I guess my own mother in a sense was very involved in the community and I think that's probably where I drew most of my desire from." A number of those interviewed spoke of their involvement in grassroots campaigning for local, state, and national legislators through phone calls and letter-writing, door-to-door campaigning, and the like. Others spoke of experience with writing issue papers and lobbying; still others had built grassroots organizations, for example, The Marshalltown Economic Development Impact Group of Iowa reported by Beverly Nelson-Forbes, Iowa State Legislator.

BEING A HEALTH RESOURCE

Because of their credibility, the nurses interviewed were often a health resource to the public and their colleagues. This gave them unique ways to interface with the public. They provided health care, listened to neighbors and constituents about their health concerns, helped people negotiate systems, gave compelling arguments to advance health legislation, and informed others so they could make intelligent decisions on legislation and policy. Meister (1985) said "Sound policies improve the health of the nation by improving the health of individuals. Therefore, policy development must include the best possible information about the needs of individuals and how well health care meets those needs" (p. 155). Nurses in public office and appointments are educationally prepared and in an optimum position to provide "the best possible information" to shape policy development. They use their backgrounds as practitioners, educators, and researchers to advance critical agendas.

Mel Callan ran for state senator, then county legislator in Rochester, New York. She said, "Nursing education prepares you to be a decision maker and independent thinker, to view things differently in a comprehensive manner." Marilyn Lee said she couldn't separate herself from the profession. "You're a nurse all the time; it is part of your persona. This may not be true of other professions. People tell you their life stories." In describing how her background influenced the decisions she made, Mary Moseley said, "As nurses, you are experts in health care . . . you know more than legislators about health care." Colleagues, policy makers, and other leaders consult Eddie Bernice Johnson. She said, "People feel you have a defined body of knowledge, so it carries an expectation." In her role as chief of staff, Sheila Burke was "a constant conduit of information" between and among people. Eve Franklin is very "nurse-identified" in the Montana State Legislature. She is seen as an expert in health policy. Her constituents find her if they are ill. Allison Giles used her experience with patients and families to see holes in systems that could be improved to result in better patient outcomes. Her impact has been largely at the local level, "where most things happen." Claire Shulman has been able to advance health care in Queens, New York by providing services that increase access to health care. Because of her background in nursing, she understands the need to have well-equipped hospitals, mobile vans that bring health care directly into communities, and educational health fairs. She said:

> I have a really good relationship with the people who run the hospitals . . . If they need equipment I have given money to buy equipment at both city hospitals . . . We set up an eye clinic . . . rehab . . . the ER. Queens Hospital is going to be state of the art, the best hospital in the city when it's finished.

In discussing issues she has brought to the table, Shulman felt that her focus on health care was directly related to being a nurse. "It just happens to be because I'm a nurse that I'm interested in the subject [health care] . . . I don't think anyone sitting in my chair who is not a nurse would engage in this."

NURSING SKILLS AS POLITICAL SKILLS

Mary Moseley, former aide to Senator Bill Frist (R-Tennessee), said that important skills of nurses are being nonjudgmental, looking at the whole person, and having "people skills." United States Representative Carolyn McCarthy (D-New York) said that the skill of being a woman prepared her for her role in Congress. She said, "You always deal with politics, whether its P.T.A., Little League, etc. Nursing is politics. People skills and life experience are the political skills you need." Many of those interviewed concurred that these skills are essential to public service roles. Several had backgrounds in community health or had substantial volunteer work within communities. These individuals pointed out that community skills often involve consensus-building, which is another strong political skill. Public health also gave them a perspective that put them in the forefront of political issues, for example, gun control, environmental issues, third party reimbursement, and Medicare and Medicaid legislation. Judy Robson, Wisconsin State Legislator, said that nurses have good problem solving skills, team skills, networking and coalition building skills, and people skills, all of which are used "every minute of the day." Her previous experiences with injustices in her clinical practice also gave her cause to lobby insurance companies and eventually run for the assembly in her state. Kristine Gebbie, former AIDS Policy Coordinator at The White House, said that she developed the political skills she needed throughout her career in nursing. She emphasized negotiating and balancing power as two important skills that were pervasive in her political appointment. In her experiences in the departments of health in the states of Oregon and Washington, and in her own education as a nurse she studied these skills, wrote about them in books and articles, and taught others how to develop and use the skills of negotiation and balance of power. Janegale Boyd uses her psychiatric nursing background to help her deal with the "multiple personalities in the state capitol" in Florida.

"FIRE IN THE BELLY": BEING PASSIONATE ABOUT WHAT YOU DO

A number of the nurses who were interviewed grew up during a period of great social and political change, exemplified by President John F. Kennedy's statement: "Ask not what your country can do for you; ask what you can do for your country." The mid-1960s through the early 1970s were times when the country struggled through issues of social injustice, equal rights, access to health care, space travel, and the Vietnam conflict. This was the era of the Peace Corps. Nursing as a career gave people an opportunity to give back to society, address the issues of the day, and create a better world. Paula Hollinger, Maryland State Legislator, talked about the "fire in my belly" as what spurred her on to campaigning for office. She described herself as a "political junkie," and told how she "fought" for women and children's health and against the HMOs. Christine Canavan, in describing a former Massachusetts State Representative who ran for Lieutenant Governor, also said he had "fire in his belly." She said he had a love and drive that were contagious and influenced her involvement in politics.

Susan Reinhard, Deputy Commissioner of the New Jersey Department of Health and Senior Services, said that during her years in education and health policy she has been known as "someone who worked in a 'passionate way'" in relation to the services she provided. Eddie Bernice Johnson, United States Representative from Texas, started her political career in the 1960s, when as a young woman she worked to get people out to vote in Texas. She knew that there were important things needing to be changed in society, so she got involved in civic work at first. Despite racial bias, she volunteered for a number of health-related community activities, e.g., glaucoma testing. She said that nursing gave her comfort, even in working through the "color line" of the South. Because of her passion for racial equality, she paired up with other concerned citizens to bring about change. These events in her life and the encouragement of others led her to public office.

HAVING PREVIOUS EXPOSURE TO POLITICAL BEHAVIOR

Winter and Lockhart (1997) studied 11 politically active nurses to understand their motivations and the obstacles that confronted them. Among the facilitators of political involvement were family environment and early exposure to political activities. They found that positive family environments "were conducive to debate and accepting of political and/or community participation" (p. 247). One of the participants said that her "father was the chairman of the Democratic Committee . . . and . . . we all got . . . on the bandwagon. [Also] my grandparents . . . used to argue interminably about politics . . . grandfather was a Democrat and grandmother was a Republican" (p. 247). Allison Giles believes that public service is important. Her great-grandfather was a Congressman and her parents were in the Navy. Also, living in Washington, DC gave her an opportunity to see lobbyists conduct their business. Family discussions helped her develop the skills for public service.

Having a father who was a Massachusetts State Representative for a number of years exposed Kate Malliarakis to politics at an early age. When her husband campaigned twice for the United States Congress, Lois Capps was by his side, campaigning for him, "stretching his exposure," and discussing health issues. She saw political behavior through the election process and in the early days of his administration. Marilyn Lee's husband was also in politics and had held office, and she had been active in the Democratic Party for a long time. These experiences helped her develop the political skills she needed to carry out her work in the Hawaii State Legislature. Janegale Boyd's brother-in-law became a Florida legislator and that spurred her on to seek public office in south Florida. For Barbara Wright, working at the Department of Higher Education in New Jersey taught her a lot about how public policy is made. She "saw politics from the inside," and learned what worked and what not to do.

THE PRESENCE OF MENTORS AND ROLE MODELS

Mentors can serve many purposes in developing and guiding people. Nancy Valentine and Virginia Trotter Betts both saw their mentors as people to talk with and from whom they could get honest feedback . One question asked whether or not anyone had served as a mentor in guiding or getting those interviewed to their positions. Responses were unexpectedly disparate. For example, Captain Veronica Stephens, former Chief Nurse of the Federal Bureau of Prisons and currently Consultant in the Program Development Division of the Office of Emergency Preparedness, felt she had extremely good mentors, and has tried to mentor others. Despite this, she expressed concern that more often than not "nurses eat their young." This age-old problem still persists, and acts to impede the progress of nurses, both individually and as a collective. Claiming that no nurses were mentors, and not much mentoring went on in the Maryland State Legislature, Marilyn Gold-water also said that women legislators did help her when she first took office. She said that "once elected, you learn your way around and make friends." Similarly, Beverly Nelson-Forbes said, "Nobody guided me in this position as far as the legislature is concerned."

In contrast, Eileen Cody said that Margarita Prentice, a Washington State Senator, was a mentor to her. She said, "Nurses who are elected should mentor other nurses and women." Allison Giles said that Congressman William Thomas (R-California) guid-ed her most. "He never settled for anything. He knows policies and the political environment." Paula Hollinger considered Rosalee Abrams a role model, someone who Hollinger said "broke the mold of the 'old boys game.'" Rosemary Nelson, Program Manager and Chief Information Officer for the Pacific Regional Program Office (PERPO) of the United States Department of Defense, identified a Navy Captain as a mentor, saying, "He had a different way of thinking, vertical and lateral, sideways." Cindy Empson identified the Kansas State Representative she replaced (who chose not to run for re-election) as a mentor. According to Margaret Leonard, Vice President of Clinical Services for HealthSource, who ran for political office in Nassau County, New York, her daughter had studied political science and was a men-tor to her; she was also her campaign manager.

Several people, while not able to identify a single mentor, referred to support systems consisting of colleagues, faculty, fel-low students, and family. Sheila Burke, for example, said that she valued Thelma Schorr's leadership, that Mary Anne Tuft (then Executive Director of the National Student Nurses Association) was a fine manager and executive, and that Claire Fagin and Rheba deTornyay were active in nursing organizations. These leaders were role models of behaviors that Burke found to be exemplary. For Mary Wakefield, Billye Brown continues to be someone she still feels "comfortable about picking up the phone and calling and asking 'What do you think about. . . .?'" Several mentors stood out for Shirley Chater as well. These included deans of schools where she received her bachelors and master's degrees and, when she was Vice Chancellor, the Chancellor at University of San Francisco. For Nancy McKelvey, faculty in each school she attended served as mentors, and for Bonnie Ryan it was nursing instructors, a staff development nurse in Texas, and a head nurse in Illinois. Winter and Lockhart (1997) found that role models fostered the "call" to political involvement for the individuals they interviewed:

> Both contemporary nurses and individuals prominent in the media were cited as influences that facilitated political involvement by either sharing their expertise or serving as sources of inspiration for the participants during their formative years. These mentors often assisted [with] learning the social behaviors and decision-making skills needed . . . (p. 247)

CARING ON A "GRAND SCALE"

Jean Watson's theory of nursing (Watson, 1985) focuses on caring, a humanistic perspective, and a scientific knowledge base. She makes several assumptions about caring; among these are that caring promotes health and growth and caring is practiced interpersonally. Health promotion, rather than cure of disease, is the domain of nursing. During the interviews, participants often used the term "caring," as well as "health promotion," "humanistic," and "scientifically grounded," to describe their work in the public sector. For example, Eileen Cody said that as a legislator you educate people on issues, just as you educate patients regarding their health. Eve Franklin felt that politics is an extension of the "helper role" of the nurse. Margaret Leonard described the role her nursing background played in preparing to run for office as going from a single life (caring for individuals) to "the abstract of many lives" (caring for the public). Likewise, Bonnie Ryan offered that "Nursing is caring for patients . . . team building and strategic planning are like care planning. Unique situations and people in patient care are akin to organizational change." Mary McGrattan said that there is "a lot of satisfaction in bedside nursing when you can make someone comfortable, and now, when you're able to help somebody through the maze of bureaucracy to help them with an issue."

PIONEERING EFFORTS

What also became apparent through the interview process was that there are many "firsts" that speak to the pioneer efforts of these leaders. For example, Representative Eddie Bernice Johnson (D-Texas) shared that she was the first nurse in the Texas Senate and the United States House of Representatives. As Commissioner of the Social Security Administration, The Honorable Shirley S. Chater was the first nurse appointed to a Cabinet level position in the federal government. Representative Paula Hollinger (D-Maryland State Legislator) said she was the first nurse legislator to create a transition program for 2- and 3-year nursing graduates that became a model program for other states. Although not interviewed for the book, Dr. Carolyne Davis, in her role as HCFA (Health Care Financing Administration) Administrator, was instrumental in implementing DRGs (Diagnostic Related Groups) (Berkowitz, 1995). Nancy Valentine, Assistant Chief and Medical Director of Nursing Programs in the Department of Veterans Affairs, established the first national distance learning program through the Uniformed Services University.

Susan Reinhard, Deputy Commissioner of the Department, New Jersey Department of Health and Senior Services, is the first nurse in New Jersey to hold this position. This department was created by the Governor in response to Reinhard's idea to combine senior services into one department. Kate Malliarakis became a nurse practitioner in 1976, when the role was first being defined. She participated in founding two of the early nurse practitioner organizations (Alliance for Nurse Practitioners and the College of Nurse Practitioners). Becoming a nurse practitioner was a real turning point for her to look "beyond the box." Carolyn McCarthy reported that she was the first woman elected to New York's 4th Congressional District.

As we begin the 21st century, it is safe to say that the fourth stage of political activism, "leading the way," is firmly in place and "making a difference" is taking hold. The chapters that follow provide evidence of how, by leading the way, nurses have been able to make a difference. To advance the notion of leading and making a difference, the book continues with a perspective on who led us before, who leads us today, the impact of nurses as a social force, and how to develop the skills and strategies that support the capability of nurses who have an interest in and/or intent to seek public positions.

REFERENCES

An interview with Mary K. Wakefield, PhD, RN, FAAN. (1992). *Healthcare Trends & Transition, 3*(6), 14–17.

Backer, B. A., Costello-Nikitas, D., Mason, D. J., McBride, A. B., & Vance, C. (1993). Power at the policy table: When women and nurses are involved. *Revolution: The Journal of Nurse Empowerment, 3,* 68–76.

Berkowitz, E. (1995). HCFA oral history interview: Interview of Carolyne Davis in her office in Washington, DC, on 8 November 1995. Available online: http://www.ssa.gov/search97.

Betts, V. T. (1996). Nursing's Agenda for Health Care Reform: Policy, politics, and power through professional leadership. *Nursing Administration Quarterly, 20*(3), 1–8.

Beverly Malone appointed to key federal position. (1999, December). American Nurses Association press release, 1–3.

Bullough, V., & Bullough, B. (1984). Nurses and power: Professional power vs. political clout. *Women & Politics, 4*(4), 67–74.

Capps, L. (1998). Nurses' voices needed in halls of congress. *American Journal of Nursing, 98*(9), 80.

Cohen, S. S., Mason, D. J., Kovner, C., Leavitt, J. K., Pulcini, J., & Sochalski, J. (1996). Stages of nursing's political development: Where we've been and where we ought to go. *Nursing Outlook, 44*(6), 259–265.

DeParle, J. (1995, Nov. 12). Sheila Burke is the militant feminist commie peacenik who's telling Bob Dole what to think. *The New York Times Magazine,* pp. 32–38, 90, 100–105.

Federici, N. (1996, May-June). Capitol chronicle: Democracy is not a spectator sport. *Washington-Nurse, 26*(3), 16–17.

Ferguson, V. (1985). Power, politics, and policy in nursing. In R. Wieczorek (Ed.), *Power, politics, and policy in nursing* (pp. 5–11). New York: Springer Publishing Co.

Gil, D. G. (1981). *Unraveling social policy* (3rd ed.). Cambridge, MA: S. Chenkman Books.

Hayes, E., & Fritsch, R. (1988). An untapped resource: The political potential of nurses. *Nursing Administration Quarterly, 13*(1), 33–39.

Lerner, H. M. (1985). In R. Wieczorek (Ed.), *Power, politics, and policy in nursing* (pp. 90–94). New York: Springer Publishing Co.

Lescavage, N. J. (1995, January/February). Nurses, make your presence felt: Taking off the rose-colored glasses. *Nursing Policy Forum, 1*(1), 18–21.

Lewenson, S. B. (1996). *Taking charge: Nursing suffrage and feminism in America, 1873–1920.* New York: National League for Nursing Press.

MacPherson, K. I. (1987). Health care policy, values, and nursing. *Advances in Nursing Science, 9*(3), 1–11.

Maraldo, P. (1985). The illusion of power. In R. Wieczorek (Ed.), *Power, politics, and policy in nursing* (pp. 64–73). New York: Springer Publishing Co.

Mason, D. J., Backer, B. A., & Georges, C. A. (1991). Toward a feminist model for the political empowerment of nursing. *Image: Journal of Nursing Scholarship, 23*(2), 72–77.

Meister, S. B. (1985, May/June). Building bridges between practice and health policy. *Maternal-Child Nursing, 10,* 155–157.

Riddle, M. (1993). In N. Birnbach & S. B. Lewenson (Eds.), *Legacy of leadership: Presidential addresses from the Superintendents' Society and the National League of Nursing Education, 1894–1952* (p. 84). New York: National League for Nursing Press. (Originally published 1911).

Robson, J. B. (1998). One nurse's journey to becoming a policymaker. In D. Mason & J. K. Leavitt (Eds.), *Policy and politics in nursing and health care* (3rd ed.). Philadelphia: Saunders.

Schutzenhofer, K. K., & Cannon, S. B. (1986, March/April). Moving nurses into the political process. *Nurse Educator, 11*(2), 26–28.

SNA members appointed to federal positions. (1999, July/August). *American Nurse, 31*(4), 3.

Stevens, B. J. (1985). Nursing, politics, and policy formulation. In R. Wieczorek (Ed.), *Power, politics, and policy in nursing* (pp. 16–21). New York: Springer Publishing Co.

Terry, R. W. (1993). *Authentic leadership: Courage in action.* San Francisco: Jossey-Bass.

Watson, J. (1985). *Nursing: The philosophy and science of caring.* Boulder, CO: Colorado Associated University Press.

Winter, M. K., & Lockhart, J. S. (1997, Sept.-Oct.). From motivation to action: Understanding nurses' political involvement. *Nursing & Health Care Perspectives, 18,* 244–247.

Historical Perspective on Nurses Active in the Political Process

> The one idea I wish above all to bring out is, that among the many opportunities for civic and altruistic work pressing on all sides nurses having superior advantages in their practical training should not rest content with being only nurses, but should use their talents wherever possible in reform and civic movements.
>
> —Lillian D. Wald

POLITICAL ACTION, PROFESSIONAL GAIN

Evidence of nursing's political activity lies in the history of the modern nursing movement, dating from 1873. Nurses have a rich background of political activity (Hall-Long, 1995; Lewenson, 1996, 1998; Rogge, 1987) although they are often recalled in late 20th century literature as politically disinterested and unaware. Stories about the formation of professional organizations, the struggle for nurse registration laws, the connection of professional organizations to the woman suffrage movement, the alliances formed with the woman's movement[1] at the beginning of the 20th century, and the work of individual nurses such as Isabel Hampton Robb, Lillian Wald, Lavinia Dock, Martha Franklin, Margaret Sanger, Adah

---

[1] The term "woman's movement" refers to women's efforts toward equality during the late 19th and early 20th century, whereas women's movement refers to the political activism during second half of this century, beginning in the 1960s.

Thoms, and others emphasize the merger of public service and professional growth. With this discussion of political activism and public service comes the issue of power—power being something that harnesses the energy of nurses within the nursing profession to improve upon and make changes for the greater good. The struggle for power has followed the profession since its inception. Nurse historian and feminist Joanne Ashley (1973) poignantly noted that

> Our very history can be described as a power struggle; the struggle to obtain a proper education though opposed by more powerful groups, the struggle to throw off the burden of oppression imposed by those groups, the struggle for the freedom to practice without numerous and professionally extraneous restraints and restrictions . . . the need to convince others of the value of nursing and its place in the health care scheme. (p. 638)

Nurses have had to address opposition from hospital administrators and physicians. Nurses have had to overcome the nursism, or prejudice toward the caring role, when they have tried to recruit women into the profession and when they have tried to control its educational and practical experiences. The acceptance of nursism by the profession has in some way contributed to the disregard for nursing's history and the omission of stories of political activism from the professional literature (Lewenson, 1996, 1998). Uncovering the activity of nurses throughout the past century allows for greater interpretation of these activities, while demonstrating the need for political knowledge and awareness (Rogge, 1987).

The framework of political activism described by Cohen et al. (1996) and discussed in chapter one provides a valuable tool to study nursing's political activism in the past, and serves as a reference to where we are today. In looking at nurses who have been appointed to important positions in government, and who have held public office, in the last few years of the 20th century, we can see how many of these professionals straddle Cohen's third and fourth stages of "political sophistication" and "leading the way," respectively. Who they are, how they got there, and what they have done will be described in subsequent chapters. In this chapter, their connection to nursing's historical involvement in political activism is explored. The stages of political activity offer a point of reference from which we can look at the activism in nursing's history and tell the stories of the growth of the profession. Here we present the story of the opening of nurse's training schools in 1873, the drive to organize the profession, the need to control education and practice, the close ties with the woman's movement at the beginning of the 20th century, and the women's movement of the later part, the image of nursing, and the individuals who reflect one or all of the four stages.

OPENING OF NURSE TRAINING SCHOOLS

With the opening of Nightingale-influenced nurse training schools in the United States in 1873, the nursing profession as we know it took shape. Prior to 1873, few trained nurses existed. Women provided care in the home for their families and neighbors. Hospital nursing was confined to untrained women, often with unsavory backgrounds. Society saw nursing as women's work and, since women's work required little education, nursing shared the low social status typically accorded to women in general. Although society valued the care provided by women, women had few rights or privileges assigned to them. Women in the 19th and early 20th centuries faced major political battles in order to own property, and to be able to vote. Nurses faced similar dilemmas in their professional struggles to establish the nursing profession, necessitating a strong coalition of nurses to argue for the control of practice and education. Early nursing pioneers faced arbitrary hospital boards comprised mostly of men. These women had to learn the art of negotiation, compromise, and conciliation in order to accomplish their professional goals. They focused on wresting from the control of men what they felt rightly belonged to women in relation to controlling nursing education and practice. Following Florence Nightingale's recommendation that nursing should remain in the hands of capable women, nursing leaders organized professional associations to gain support and political clout from the increasing numbers of nursing graduates (Cook, 1913; Lewenson, 1996; "Progress and Reaction," 1908; Roberts, 1954).

ORGANIZED NURSING

By 1893, 20 years following the opening of the first Nightingale-influenced training schools at Bellevue Hospital, New Haven, and Massachusetts General, superintendents of nurse's training schools recognized a need to share their experiences and harness their collective energy. The need to standardize nursing education, and to establish collegial relationships among the superintendents was the impetus for nursing leaders, such as Linda Richards, Isabel Hampton Robb, and Lavinia Dock, to form organized professional nursing organizations. Superintendents of nurses' training schools formed the American Society of Superintendents of Training Schools for Nurses (renamed the National League of Nursing Education in 1912 and the National League for Nursing in 1952) in Chicago at the World's Fair Congress on Hospitals, Dispensaries, and Nursing.

Nursing educator Isabel Stewart (1949) described the World's Fair Congress in 1893 as the "'coming out' of nursing as a profession" (p. xv). Nurses in the United States joined other nurses from around the world to showcase their professional growth in the brief 20 years since nurses' training schools had opened. Invited by the English nursing organizer Ethel Bedford Fenwick to work on the United States exhibit, Isabel Hampton Robb organized the Nursing Congress. Robb examined the issues faced by nursing superintendents as they oversaw the nurses' training programs, and they used the Nurses' Congress as a forum to discuss these issues. Papers presented at the Congress reflected the need for a uniform curriculum; the need to lengthen the curriculum from 1 or 2 years to 3 years; the need to address problems related to the opening of an increasing number of nurses' training schools that served the financial needs of the hospital, rather than the educational needs of the student; and the desire for the protection that nurses' registration would afford them (Benson, 1993).

Eighteen superintendents gathered at the World's Fair and established one of the first professional organizations for nurses. Sophia Palmer (1897/1991) believed that "Organization is the power of the day. Without it nothing great is accomplished" (p. 297). Palmer saw the need to harness the energy of nurses who graduated from the newly opened training schools. In 1880, 15 schools of nursing had graduated 157 trained nurses. In 1890, 35 schools were open, graduating 471 trained nurses. In 1900, the numbers had increased dramatically to 432 schools, graduating 3,456 trained nurses (Burgess, 1928). These 18 superintendents felt a compelling need to organize in order to address the social issues of the day. In later years, Stewart (1948) remembered how they had heeded the call "To advance we must unite" (p. xvii). These extraordinary women directed their political energies to establish a new profession and to make a significant social contribution.

Nursing was considered a new profession, an opportunity for women to support themselves financially in a meaningful occupation. Franklin North wrote about this in 1883 in an article published in the popular illustrated magazine, *The Century,* entitled, "A New Profession for Women." In his story he described the nurses' training school that had opened at Bellevue Hospital. Prior to the opening of the school in 1873, patients experienced low standards of care. In 1872, however, the Local Visiting Committee of the New York State Charities Aid Association visited Bellevue and judged that the inferior care could only be addressed by trained nurses. They argued their case for the establishment of a school for nursing, and, in many instances, met resistance from physicians. The resistance grew from social, political, and professional reasons. North (1883) wrote that arguments such as the following were given in opposition to opening training schools. "The patients are of a class so difficult to deal with, and the service is so laborious, that the conscientious, intelligent women you are looking for will lose heart and hope long before the two years of training are over" (p. 39).

The training school at Bellevue was seen as a success, and the opposition expressed toward it eventually diminished. Student nurses, originally confined to one unit, were welcomed onto others. The students improved the quality of patient care and made the hospital stay more bearable. Early nursing leader Linda Richards described in her presidential address at the Second Annual Meeting of the American Society of Superintendents of Training Schools for Nurses (Superintendents' Society) how hospitals had changed significantly as a result of nurses' training schools (1895/1993).

How vastly different are the hospitals of today from those same hospitals a score of years ago! Visit Bellevue, Blackwell's Island,

Tewksbury, and many others. They all tell the same story. The perfect cleanliness and order of the yards, the homelike appearance, the contented faces of the patients, make even hospital workers wonder how so much can have been done. (p. 19)

Nursing leader and suffrage activist Lavinia Dock (1949) delivered a paper, 2 years prior to Richard's address, where she described the relationship of nurses' training schools to hospitals. Dock explained that these schools were established by women who were in "hospitals that needed them most but want them least—the city or county hospitals, where local politics grow at the expense of the neglected sick poor . . ." (p. 14). Dock understood the political nature of the work of the nursing leaders who led the early nurses' training schools. Without the ability to vote or hold political office, they had to argue their cases before hospital boards, and fought to establish nurses' training schools. Hospital administrators saw the economic advantages that a nurses' training school brought to the hospital. Very often, schools opened with little regard to the educational value that institutions could offer to the student (Roberts, 1954). Once students graduated, hospitals had little use for them. Graduates had to look elsewhere for work, and hired themselves out as private duty nurses or as visiting nurses. Hospitals used the students as staff, often shortchanging their lectures and their training. Between 1873 and 1893, little could be done or was done to control this problem. Once the Superintendents' Society had formed, however, a political mechanism to control their profession had been established.

The nurses who started the Superintendents' Society focused their political energies on establishing the profession. They fit into what Cohen et al. (1996) considered the first stage of political involvement, the "buy-in" stage. Although Cohen equates this stage to nursing in the 1970s, the case can be made that as early as the 1890s, through the establishment of their professional associations, nurses recognized the relationship and the importance of their work to political activism (Lewenson, 1998).

Also established were organizations for new graduates of training schools. Recognizing that nurses worked outside of a structured setting and had little opportunity to meet together, the founders of the Superintendents' Society encouraged the formation of alumnae associations at each training school. Alumnae associations provided the graduate-trained nurse with a connection to other nurses. In some cases, the alumnae associations offered a nurses' directory that assisted the nurse to secure private duty positions. In 1897, Sophia Palmer, first editor of the *American Journal of Nursing (AJN)*, presented the results of a survey on the development of alumnae associations. She noted that the object of most alumnae associations was for the:

> union of the graduates of respective schools, for mutual help and protection; to promote social intercourse and good fellowship; to provide friendly and pecuniary assistance in times of illness or death among members, and to advance the interest of the nursing profession. (Palmer, 1897/1991, p. 294)

The Superintendents' Society encouraged the development of these smaller associations, believing that they could be used as a mechanism to organize the next professional organization to form the Nurses Associated Alumnae of the United States and Canada (renamed the American Nurses Association in 1911) (Dock, 1896/1991a). The idea behind organizing the smaller alumnae associations reflected the need for collective action. In order to control the education and practice of the profession, a united front was essential. Palmer (1897/1991) noted that "all questions having ultimate advancement of the profession are dependent upon united action for success" (p. 297). Organization of these early graduates into this second professional nursing organization became an important goal of the Superintendents' Society. A committee of 12 members met at their second convention in 1895 to organize this group.

After reviewing the structure of several other professional and governmental organizations, Dock (1896/1991a) recommended that the Nurses Associated Alumnae be organized through the alumnae associations of each school. These smaller associations would join state associations that would ultimately join a larger national association. The Superintendents' Society liked Dock's plan, and met with a delegation from 12 alumnae associations in 1896 to write a constitution for the new organization. Members of the Superintendents' Society approved the formation of this new association in 1897. The following year, the Nurses' Associated

Alumnae held its first convention in New York State. At that first meeting held in 1898, 23 nurse alumnae associations already existed and joined. The number dramatically increased to 142 alumnae associations in 1912. Nurses were ready and willing to join and participate in the professional organizations.

The architects of this new professional organization saw the connection between their professional aspirations and their political involvement, consonant with the stage of political activism (Cohen et al., 1996). For example, nursing leaders were concerned about the fact that anyone could call himself or herself a nurse. They felt the need to protect the public from unscrupulous people practicing nursing, as well as to protect the professional, who was confronted with unwanted competition from the untrained nurse. Registration laws became one of the major issues that were addressed early by the Nurses Associated Alumnae and that required political strategies to change. Nurses had to argue their cases before elected officials, while still not having the vote. Much skill was required to gain the support of legislators without being able to offer them their vote. One of the reasons given in 1908 by some nurses for not supporting a resolution to support woman suffrage was their fear of alienating some of the legislators against them because they needed their vote for state registration. In a letter to the *AJN* in 1908, nurse Edith Thuresson Kelly wrote how nurses enjoyed the benefits of the political battle waged by the woman's movement. She felt, however, that entering the political struggle for suffrage would have to wait until nurses had obtained state registration (Lewenson, 1996). Louise Croft Boyd (1908) also cautioned the readers of the *AJN* not to confront men and legislators about woman suffrage, saying that they "would quickly side against a nurse registration law which was pushed forward by women who were also working in favor of equal suffrage" (p. 136).

During the struggle for nurse registration laws, nurses learned how to prepare bills, seeking the expert advice of lawyers. They also sought support from other women's groups, such as the National Council of Women; wrote about the issue; and published articles in professional journals and lay magazines (Birnbach, 1985). Nurses clearly saw the relationship between political activism and the advancement of the nursing profession. The first four nurse registration laws were passed in 1903 in North Carolina,

New Jersey, New York, and Virginia. By 1923, nurses and the public in 48 states had some form of legal protection afforded by a state nurse registration law. Due to the inexperience of the nurses in arguing for nurse registration, many of the laws were inadequate, and required even greater skill in changing them (Roberts, 1954).

The next two nursing organizations to form were the National Association of Colored Graduate Nurses (NACGN) in 1908 and the National Organization of Public Health Nurses (NOPHN) in 1912. Both groups organized to serve the needs of special groups in nursing. The NACGN organized to meet the concerns of African American nurses, who, depending on their state, were excluded from membership in the Nurses Associated Alumnae because of racial prejudice and, subsequently, from the American Nurses Association. To address the concerns for control of education and practice in addition to the racism that these nurses experienced, African American nurses organized the NACGN. Martha Franklin, one of the founders of this group, recognized the need to organize her colleagues in order to make changes in nursing and in racial status (Carnegie, 1991; Hine, 1989). This organization had few connections to the Superintendents' Society or the Nurses Associated Alumnae; however; it shared close ties with the newly formed NOPHN (Lewenson, 1996).

The NOPHN organized for the protection, control, and advancement of public health nursing. The very nature of public health forced nurses to become politically engaged, that is, they recognized the close connection between political persuasion and improvement of the health of the public. Lillian Wald, for example, one of the founders of the NOPHN, and her colleague, Mary Brewster established the Henry Street Settlement in the Lower East Side of New York City in 1893. There they witnessed the deleterious effect of poverty, overcrowding, poor working conditions, and inadequate sanitation on families in the community. Appalled by these conditions, Wald and Brewster moved into the neighborhood and opened one of the first nurses' settlement houses. The Henry Street Settlement became a hotbed of political activism for the public health nurses who worked there.

In keeping with the interests of other social reformers during the late 1800s, Wald and her peers related the health problems within the community to the untoward social, economic, and political conditions that existed. One of the many examples of Wald's political accomplishments was the inclusion of public health nurses in the public schools. Following a brief experiment in 1902 that demonstrated the value of a nurse in a public school, Wald persuaded public officials to hire Lina Rogers as a school nurse. In doing so Wald "connected her caring with activism by initiating practice and policy changes via administrative and organizational skills, persuasiveness, coalitions, delivering testimony and political power" (Backer, 1993, p. 128).

Lavinia Dock, Wald's friend and colleague, moved into the Henry Street Settlement and spent 20 years living among other social reformers and public health nurses. In doing so, she found a cadre of like-minded individuals who saw nursing's social obligation and commitment to the public. These women worked together and shared in the day-to-day concerns about patient care as well as the affairs of the world at large. They supported the rights of women and lobbied for peace. Engaged in the neighborhood's political community, they shared the other struggles being waged at the time. Concern for unfair labor practice, tenement house reform, and child labor legislation all involved the nurses at Henry Street. This strong affinity of the nurse to social obligation and responsibility became the hallmark of public health nursing.

The value of public health nurses spread, and visiting nurse services opened throughout the country. By 1890, 21 visiting nurse organizations existed and by 1905, the number had increased to over 171 (Fitzpatrick, 1975; Gardner, 1933). This service rapidly spread to more and more cities. Fearing that too many visiting nurse organizations were being controlled by those who were unconcerned about nursing standards, public health nursing leaders such as Wald and others believed that a new organization was needed.

Lack of common standards, educational requirements, or connection among these visiting nurse services, and a need to set public health nursing care standards prompted the formation of the NOPHN in 1912 (Fitzpatrick, 1975; Gardner, 1933). The NOPHN focused their efforts on increasing interest in public health nursing, establishing ethical and technical standards of care, facilitating the joint efforts of those interested in public health in the community, and creating a central clearinghouse for information about public health nursing (Fitzpatrick, 1975).

TIES TO THE WOMAN'S MOVEMENT

The new profession of nursing attracted middle-class women who before 1873 had few, if any opportunities to earn their own livelihood. Most women became wives or stayed at home to care for relatives. These new training schools for nursing provided women with an education and skill that they could use to financially support themselves. Stewart (1948) wrote that training schools gave women a chance to become useful outside of the "domestic sphere, emancipating them and giving them a chance to grow" (p. 78).

Women were attracted to the nursing profession at a time when progressive ideas about social reform captured the imagination of the American public. Politically minded citizens showed concern for exploitation of the worker, indiscriminant use of child labor, increasing numbers of immigrants in cities, and the problems of overcrowded conditions that they brought. Benson (1993) refers to the 1890s, the last decade of the 19th century, as a time of great social change and social unrest. The nursing profession allowed women to leave the safety of their assigned roles as wives and housekeepers and offered them an opportunity to apply their talents to a professional role.

With the organization of nursing's four professional associations, nurses gained an important power base. Dock (1904/1991b) noted with some chagrin, however, that the Superintendents' Society rarely used or recognized the latent power they had in public work. Dock wrote:

> Yet this Society, as one body, would often be astonished at the actual extent and weight of its influence, if its whole latent and, at present unsuspected power, were actually to be systematically exerted in an intelligent and energetic manner. (p. 320)

Dock constantly reminded nurses of their social and political obligations to support social reforms, particularly woman suffrage. She equated suffrage with the ability of nurses to provide quality patient care and improve the human condition for the families for which they cared. Her numerous articles on the subject, published in the *AJN* and the few other nursing journals that existed at the time, spread her ideas to trained nurses and nursing educators. In 1907, Dock was already advising the nursing readership of the *AJN* about the importance of woman suffrage for the profession and why nurses needed to expand their world-views. She knew that a large majority of nurses focused solely on their work, maintaining a parochial outlook. Nurses and the nursing organizations they formed were engaged in tending nursing issues and concerns. Dock (1907) argued, however, that nursing had to look outward toward larger issues in order to further both the profession and the health of their patients. She wrote:

> As the modern nursing movement is emphatically an outcome of the original and general woman movement and as nurses are no longer a dull, uneducated class, but an intelligent army of workers, capable of continuous progress, and fitted to comprehend the idea of social responsibility, it would be a great pity for them to allow one of the most remarkable movements of the day to go on under their eyes without comprehending it. (pp. 896–897)

Dock encouraged the state associations to continue their efforts for state registration, support of trained nurses, and the promotion of ethical standards. She hoped, however, that the national nursing associations would support the social and political movements of the day. She reasoned that because modern life was so interwoven, organized nursing could no longer stay uninvolved and "yet demand the interest and the respect of society as a whole for ourselves and our individual problems" (Dock, 1907, p. 899). When the Nurses' Alumnae Association failed to vote to support a suffrage resolution in 1908, Dock became even more committed to raising the level of awareness of organized nursing (Lewenson, 1996). Undaunted by the initial failure in 1908 to gain the Nurses' Associated Alumnae support for woman suffrage, Dock (1908) wrote, "I cannot see why a nurse should forget that she is a citizen, and a citizen who owes a great number of her advantages to the women pioneers who have fought the women's fight (p. 366)."

Dock (1908) urged nurses in both the Superintendents' Society and the Nurses' Associated Alumnae to join with other women's groups already engaged in the suffrage movement. Both organizations pooled their resources and formed the American Federation of Nurses in 1901 to enable groups to become part of the National Council of Women, and ultimately, the International Council of Women (Lewenson, 1996). The American Federation of Nursing existed between 1901 and 1912, when the Nurses Associated Alumnae changed its name to the American Nurses Association (ANA) and took on the responsibility of representing organized nursing abroad (Lewenson, 1996). Through a national and international connection with these women's groups, nurses surpassed Cohen's Stage One, since some moved onto Stages Two (self-interest) and Three (political sophistication) by participating in and involving themselves with the political issues that women universally addressed.

Lavinia Dock, Adelaide Nutting (nursing educator and President of the American Federation of Nursing), and others increased their efforts to educate nurses about woman suffrage and linked all kinds of health promotion and prevention measures to obtaining the vote. For example, they argued, without the vote, nurses would be able neither to serve their public nor to further reform, either within the profession or outside it. Political activism was in the form of educating nursing and the public to the relevance of suffrage and good health. Annie Damer, President of the Nurses' Associated Alumnae in 1909, advocated preparation of nursing students with the idea of civic responsibility and encouraged students to practice self-government while in school (Lewenson, 1996). Damer (1909) addressed her colleagues with great passion, saying, "When you are asked to begin work for enfranchisement of women, begin it right at home" (p. 904). In 1912, Dock and many other nursing leaders gained the support for an organizational suffrage resolution that would send four delegates from the newly formed American Federation of Nursing, to the International Council of Nursing meeting, where women throughout the world were voting to support woman suffrage (Ashley, 1976; Chinn, 1985; Lewenson, 1996; Wheeler, 1985). Pleased with the vote, Dock continued her efforts to persuade the members of her profession to support the suffrage effort until it was finally won in 1920.

NURSING AND THE MODERN WOMEN'S MOVEMENT

Organized nursing maintained close ties with the woman's movement of the first part of the 20th century; however, its relationship with the second wave of feminism did not initially fare as well. Feminists in the 1960s found themselves struggling with preconceived, devalued notions of women's work. They sought to break down barriers to gain entry into traditionally male professions, such as law and medicine. The outcome of this tension often downplayed the traditional women's professions in favor of the financially and socially valued work of men.

In challenging the traditional role of the woman as wife, mother, and homemaker, feminists often overlooked the value of child-rearing or the importance of caring. With good reason, many challenged the roadblocks established by the proverbial "old boys network," and argued for equal opportunity on all fronts. Women in the 1960s had had the vote for over 40 years, but still were not in agreement about political issues, such as the Equal Rights Amendment; nor were women in agreement about expected roles of women in work, family, or community. Similar to the feminist's quest to uncover a "hidden" women's history, the nursing literature encouraged nurses to reclaim their history. Included in this search for the past is a search for who the collective "woman" is. Using a feminist perspective to examine women and nursing means that different ideas, previously omitted, become a valuable part of the history. For example, studying a woman's diary or the stories she tells her children provides insights about women that were never captured in traditional histories that looked at official documents to narrate the story. Using a feminist perspective encourages the study of the past—not to romanticize it, but to develop greater insights (Chinn & Wheeler, 1985). Social, political, economic, and intellectual commentary on nursing history revealed the source of nurses' struggles with their own equality in the world around them. They found that the political savvy of early pioneer leaders was lost to later generations of nurses, and the tools to do so had gone as well. Chinn and Wheeler (1985) noted that nursing's presence in the feminist movement of the 1960s remained "obscure" and "notably absent" (p. 74). Organized nursing remained aloof during this period, and an "uneasy" relationship formed with the feminist movement (Allen, 1985). Nursing seemed to avoid radical feminist activities, while avid feminists avoided a profession that was so closely aligned with women's work (Allen, 1985; Lewenson, 1998). When describing the similarity of the issues confronting women and nurses, McBride (1976) wrote, "Nursing is the oldest, most honorable female profession and it is saddled with just about all the problems that women see in themselves as their consciousnesses are raised" (p. 756). Changes in women's roles mirror society's perceptions of nursing roles. As women in the second half of the twentieth century challenged their inequality and sought political power, nurses did so as well.

Recognizing the shared issues between women and the nursing profession, not all nurses eschewed the feminist movement. For many, nursing roles of caregiver, advocate, teacher, and activist coincided with the social and political goals of feminists and other reform efforts of the 1960s and 1970s. According to Wilma Scott Heide (1973), nurse and President of the National Organization of Women (NOW) between 1970 and 1974, "Nursing suffers from the same oppression, prejudices, and limitations as women in our society" (p. 824). She further noted that "the status of women is tragically reflected in the status of nurses" (p. 824). Nurses needed to embrace the goals of the women's movement and find support for many of the same issues. The characteristics deplored by society and many of the feminists were some of the same characteristics that nurses valued. Traits like caring, nurturing, compassion, tenderness, submissiveness, passivity, subjectivity, and emotionalism found their way into both the woman's role and the professional role of nurses. While many of the traits made a nurse good at her or his job, some prevented them from taking a more proactive political stand. Heide (1973) urged nursing to work with the feminists in addressing the inequities in society.

Other nurses, like the noted nurse historian and feminist JoAnn Ashley (1976), argued for nurses to advocate on behalf of their patients and consumer health. Nurses needed to approach health care from a proactive political stance, knowing that there would be turf issues and power struggles to address. Ashley (1976) wrote:

> Professional nursing must begin exerting open and public leadership in meeting consumer health needs. Dominant influences in health care will not yield to the private and quiet pleas of pacifying women; powerful, male-dominated groups, economically motivated, will not be reasonable with their interests and status threatened.

Nurses must change their own attitudes toward themselves and their role. (p. 133)

By the 1970s, organized nursing had begun to respond to the support of this second wave of feminism. The ANA supported the Equal Rights Amendment, established the Nurses Coalition for Action in Politics, and organized a group called Nurses-NOW. By the 1980s, a growing acceptance of women's roles on the part of feminists became more evident. Nursing, too, began to incorporate the language of empowerment and political equality in educational curricular and professional literature. Recognition of nursing's strong ties to women's issues throughout the 21st century became more openly discussed (Allen, 1985; Andrist, 1988; Heide, 1973, 1985; McBride, 1976; Starr, 1974; Talbott & Vance, 1981). Feminist theory also found a place in nursing research and discussion. Diers (1984) wrote that nursing had become a metaphor for the "struggle of women for equality" (p. 23). Feminism, explained by Chinn and Wheeler (1985) offered "a world view that values women and that confronts systematic injustices based on gender" (p. 74), and paved the way for nurses interested in controlling their own personal and professional lives. Recognizing that change for the nursing profession and for patients could not be gained by remaining subordinate or accepting a subservient role, political strategies became part of the culture of the evolving feminist nurse. The feminist movement of the latter half of the 20th century has helped to remove some of the barriers to nursing, fostering equity with other health professionals in providing quality health care to all citizens. It has facilitated nursing's move through the political stages of development, as has been described by Cohen et al. (1996). Through acceptance of the tenets of feminism, nursing has been freer to challenge the typically patriarchal systems in health care. Being aware of the constraints nursing as a profession faces, allows for the chance to develop better strategies to combat prejudice that ultimately inhibits a better and more holistic health care system. Furthermore, and perhaps more importantly, feminism has created new models for leadership that include a different way of setting and achieving political agendas. More inclusive, and reliant on consensus-building strategies, nursing has engaged in different ways of knowing and doing (Chinn, 1995).

Well aware of the importance of the image of nursing in influencing who entered the profession, the economic and social value placed on the work of nurses, and the educational advancement of nurses, nursing has attempted to address concerns about status and image over time. Nursing's self-interest in starting and protecting the profession at the beginning of the 20th century led to nurses' involvement in legislative changes to protect their status as professionals and as women. Moreover, nurses recognized the strong connection between politics and health, and lobbied to change legislation that affected the health of their patients. Yet nurses' image as subservient doctor's handmaidens, primarily female, has persisted into the late 20th century. The image of the nurse as seen by the public has not yet caught up with much of the work that nurses throughout the century have done. Nurses themselves know little of who their political activists were and, for the most part, have done little to value or preserve their heritage. One step in increasing political activism among nurses has been nursing's study of its own history and contributions to the political landscape. Another step is the sharing in the political activism of others involved in the feminist movement. Society's views of women are reflected in its views of nurses. Little attention has been paid to the role of women and nurses in political activism. We have begun to uncover the stories of women in politics as a way of encouraging others to follow suit.

ELECTED AND APPOINTED IN HISTORY

Until 1920, women could not vote. In most instances they could not hold office. When they could hold office they could not find enough votes to support them as candidates. In the late 1800s and early 1900s, appointments to key governmental positions or local boards of health were difficult to obtain, regardless of the nurse's expertise. Legislators rarely appointed women to boards because they preferred to give those positions to people who could vote for them. Nurses at the sixth annual convention of the Superintendents' Society heard member Emma Maud Banfield (1900) explain how legislators did not want to throw away their votes on women. Organized nursing discussed the importance of political activism in order to change the social order and improve health care in this country. The struggle for nurse registration laws taught nurses how to effectively lobby for legislative change, and many nurses became involved at the local and state levels (Lewenson, 1996).

Documentation of nurses' efforts to run for public office is rare. In reviewing historical documents, the names of elected nurses prior to 1920 were not found. Although it is possible that in some local communities a nurse may have been elected to public office, a search of the literature did not reveal this information. Only one name, Margaret Brydon Laird, came to light after asking members through the American Association of the History of Nursing (AAHN) website. Nurse historian Janet Fickeissen rescued Laird's accomplishment from obscurity.

In 1920, Laird won a position in the New Jersey State Assembly. She was the first woman and first nurse to hold public office in New Jersey. Laird graduated nurses training from Newark City Hospital in 1895. She married, had two children, and maintained active membership in many women's organizations. Her own family background was steeped in political activism. Fickeissen (2000) describes Laird's mother as "a contemporary of Susan B. Anthony" who had been active in the suffrage movement. Laird's maternal grandfather, an Episcopal minister, was an active voice in the woman's rights movement as well. Laird's background led her to become actively involved in the suffrage movement. Laird accepted positions as secretary of the Essex County (NJ) Suffrage Association, chair for Newark's chapter of the National American Woman's Suffrage Association, and vice-president of the Women's Political Union. She worked on the suffrage campaign until its successful passage in 1920. Laird picketed the White House and, according to an interview done in 1968 when Laird was 97 years of age, she said that "she was disappointed she wasn't arrested" (Morgan, 1968, p. 10). Laird brought several important political issues to the table. She had sponsored a bill on prohibition early in her tenure in the legislature; however, she also supported more liberal legislation, for example, equal pay for women employed by the state, and the establishment of juvenile courts. Laird served two terms and declined from running for a third because of the late evening hours of the assembly.

Also through the efforts of Janet Fickeissen, we uncovered the name of Eloise Nagel, mayor of Shrewsbury Township, New Jersey between 1972 and 1973. Her obituary described her as a registered nurse who had retired from the Navesink House in Red Bank, New Jersey, in 1984 (Obituary, 1999). She was active in community service during World War II and continued in many civic activities throughout the 40 years that followed. She was elected in 1968 as a Democrat on the Township Committee and was "the first woman to hold an elected office in the Township's 300 year history" (Obituary, 1999).

Close in time to Nagel's political tenure, noted nurse theorist Imogene King served as alderman of her town of Wood Dale, Illinois. She recognized a need to improve the health of her community and quickly made her voice heard in the political arena. She ran for public office, one of the first women in her community to do so, faced "dirty politics" and people who were opposed to her candidacy on the basis of gender. She was able to gain support to make changes that affected the financial viability of her town, as well as the health care of some of the city workers. For example, when a police officer had a coronary she went to the chief of police and said, "we're going to do something about this." She was instrumental in starting an exercise program and instituted other preventive measures, improving the health of these employees. Through her work on the city council, council members came to recognize that nurses were smart decision makers who could solve problems.

Nursing has a strong history of political activism that spans the 20th century. This involvement in politics is chronicled by the opening of training schools, the organization of professional nursing associations, the concern of public health nurses for the health and well-being of people, participation in the suffrage movement, ties with the woman suffrage and women's movements, and the appointment of nurses and their election to political office. Each story builds upon the previous one, and, when woven together, indicates a strong sense of political awareness and growth over time. In the next chapter, we begin to tell the contemporary stories of the nurses we interviewed who have run for a public office, or been elected or appointed. We begin by describing who these leaders are, what brought them to the eye of the public, and how they have been "leading the way."

REFERENCES

Allen, M. (1985). Women, nursing and feminism: An interview with Alice J. Baumgart, RN, PhD. *Canadian Nurse, 81*(1), 20–22.

Andrist, L. (1988). A feminist framework for graduate education in women's health. *Journal of Nursing Education, 27*(2), 66–70.

Ashley, J. A. (1973). About power in nursing. *Nursing Outlook, 21*(10), 637–641.

Ashley, J. (1976). *Hospitals, paternalism and the role of the nurse.* New York: Teachers College Press.

Backer, B. (1993). Lillian Wald: Connecting caring with actions. *Nursing and Health Care, 14*(3), 122–129.

Banfield, E. M. (1900). *Sixth Annual Convention of the American Society of Superintendents' of Training Schools for Nurses.* Harrisburg, PA: Harrisburg Publishing Co.

Benson, E. (1993). Toward social reform, 1894-1913. In N. Birnbach & S. B. Lewenson (Eds.), *Legacy of leadership: Presidential addresses from the Superintendents' Society and the National League of Nursing Education* (pp. 3–14). New York: National League for Nursing Press.

Birnbach, N. (1985). Vignette: Political activism and the registration movement. In D. Mason & S. W. Talbott (Eds.), *Political action handbook for nurses: Changing the workplace, government, organizations, and community.* Menlo Park, CA: Addison-Wesley.

Boyd, L. C. (1908). The suffrage, another view. [Letter to the editor]. *American Journal of Nursing, 9*(2), 136.

Burgess, M. A. (1928). *Nurses, patients, and pocketbooks.* New York: Committee on the Grading of Nursing Schools.

Carnegie, M. (1991). *The path we tread: Blacks in nursing, 1854–1990.* New York: National League for Nursing Press.

Chinn, P. (1985). Historical roots: Female nurses and political action. *Journal of the New York Nurses Association, 16*(2), 29–37.

Chinn, P. L., & Wheeler, C. E. (1985). Feminism and nursing: Can nursing afford to remain aloof from the women's movement? *Nursing Outlook, 33*(2), 74–76.

Cohen, S. S., Mason, D. J., Kovener, C., Leavitt, J. K., Pulcini, J., & Sochalsik, J. (1996). Stages of nursing's political development: Where we've been and where we ought to go. *Nursing Outlook, 44*(6), 259–266.

Cook, E. (1913). *The life of Florence Nightingale.* London: Macmillan.

Damer, A. (1909). Presidential address. Twelfth Annual Convention of the Nurses' Associated Alumnae. *American Journal of Nursing, 9*(12), 904.

Diers, D. (1984). To profess: To be a professional. *Journal of the New York State Nurses Association, 15*(4), 23.

Dock, L. L. (1949). Relation of training schools to hospitals. In I. A. Hampton (Ed.), *Nursing of the sick 1893* (pp. 12–24). New York: McGraw-Hill (Original work published 1893)

Dock, L. L. (1991a). A national association for nurses and its legal organization. In N. Birnbach & S. B. Lewenson (Eds.), *First words: Selected addresses from the National League for Nursing 1894–1933* (pp. 298–314). New York: National League for Nursing Press. (Original work published 1896)

Dock, L. L. (1991b). The duty of this society in public work. In N. Birnbach & S. B. Lewenson (Eds.), *First words: Selected address from the National League for Nursing 1894–1933* (pp. 319–321). New York: National League for Nursing Press. (Original work published 1904).

Dock, L. L. (1907). Some urgent social claims. *American Journal of Nursing, 7,* 895–901.

Dock, L. L. (1908 August). The letter-box. *Nurses' Journal of the Pacific Coast, 4,* 366.

Eloise Nagel, 84, ex-mayor, nurse. (1999, November 26). *Asbury Park Press,* p. C8.

Fickeissen, J. L. (2000). Margaret Brydon Laird. *American nursing: A biological dictionary.* New York: Springer Publishing Co.

Fitzpatrick, M. L. (1975). *The National Organization for Public Health Nursing, 1912–1952.* New York: National League for Nursing.

Gardner, M. S. (1933). *Public health nursing* (2nd ed.) New York: Macmillan.

Hall-Long, B. A. (1995). Nursing's past, present, and future political experiences. *Nursing & Health Care: Perspectives on Community, 16*(1), 24–28.

Heide, W. S. (1973). Nursing and women's liberation: A parallel. *American Journal of Nursing, 73,* 824–827.

Heide, W. S. (1985). *Feminism for the health of it.* Buffalo, NY: Margaret-daughters.

Hine, D.C. (1989). *Black women in white: Racial conflict and cooperation in the nursing profession, 1890–1950.* Bloomington: Indiana University Press.

Lewenson, S. B. (1996). *Taking charge: Nursing, suffrage, and feminism, 1873–1920.* New York: National League for Nursing Press.

Lewenson, S. B. (1998). Historical overview: Policy, politics, and nursing. In *Policy and politics in nursing and health care* (3rd ed., pp. 41–58). Philadelphia: W. B. Saunders.

McBride, A. (1976). A married feminist. *American Journal of Nursing, 76*(5), 754–756.

Morgan, M. (1968, August 10). First assemblywomen recalls past. *Asbury Park Press,* p. 10.

North, F. H. (1883). A new profession for women. *Century, 25,* 38–47.

Palmer, S. (1991). Training school alumnae associations. In N. Birnbach & S. B. Lewenson (Eds.), *First words: Selected addresses from the National League for Nursing 1894–1933* (pp. 291–297). New York: National League for Nursing Press. (Original work published 1897)

Progress and reaction. (1908). *American Journal of Nursing, 8,* 333–334.

Richards, L. (1993). Address of President Linda Richards. In N. Birnbach & S. B. Lewenson (Eds.). *Legacy of leadership: Presidential addresses from the Superintendents' Society and the National League of Nursing Education 1894–1952* (pp. 16–19). New York: National League for Nursing Press. (Originally published 1895).

Roberts, M. M. (1954). *American nursing history and interpretation.* New York: Macmillan.

Rogge, M. M. (1987). Nursing and politics: A forgotten legacy. *Nursing Research, 36*(1), 26–30.

Starr, D. (1974). Poor baby: The nurse and feminism. *Canadian Nurse, 70*(3), 20–23.

Stewart, I. M. (1948). *The education of nurses: Historical foundations and modern trends.* New York: Macmillan.

Stewart, I. M. (1949). Introduction. In I. A. Hampton (Ed.), *Nursing of the sick, 1893* (pp. xv–xix). New York: McGraw-Hill.

Talbott, S., & Vance, C. (1981). Involving nursing in a feminist group— NOW. *Nursing Outlook, 29*(10), 592–595.

Wald, L. D. (1991). Work of women in municipal affairs. In N. Birnbach & S. B. Lewenson (Eds.), *First words: Selected addresses from the National League for Nursing 1894–1933* (pp. 315–318). New York: National League for Nursing Press. (Original work published 1900)

Wheeler, C. (1985). The *American Journal of Nursing* and the socialization of a profession. *Advances in Nursing Science, 7*(2), 20–34.

Nurses in the Political Arena:
The Face the Public Sees

> We will meet the need of the public and of the individual
> because it is our responsibility to meet the present need,
> just as it was our predecessor's to meet that of the past.

> —S. Lillian Clayton

WHO IS THE NURSE IN A PUBLIC POSITION?

In 1996 Summers wrote: "There are over 2.2 million nurses in the
United States. This means that 1 out of every 100 adults is a nurse.
One in every 44 female voters is a nurse" (p. 37). Precise findings
from the National Sample Survey of Registered Nurses—March
1996 (Findings, 1997) are that there were 2,558,874 registered
nurses (2,115,815 were employed) in 1996, the most recent data
published on the RN work force. Nurses are the largest group of
health care providers and a potentially powerful force in the public arena. Although well over 100 nurses hold federal and state
elected office, this represents a very small proportion (.005%) of
the total nursing population. These nurses are appointed to federal and state positions, serve as legislators and cabinet members in departments of health, veterans' affairs, and the uniformed
services, and other offices. For example, at the time of this writing two Congressional Fellows in the office of Senator Daniel K.
Inouye of Hawaii had been nurses. A nurse has served as Legislative
Director in the Office of Senator Patrick Moynihan of New York. A
nurse has been a legislative assistant to Senator Jeff Bingaman of
New Mexico. As of the November 1998 election, six legislators in
New Hampshire, five legislators in Connecticut and Maryland, and

four legislators in the states of Maine, Washington, and Montana are nurses. Twenty additional states were identified as having nurse legislators in 1998, making the total count at least 32 states. Research on nurses active in the political arena is scarce. "Therefore, it remains important to understand what 'calls' those nurses who do take an active role to become immersed in the process" (Winter & Lockhart, 1997, p. 246).

The 45 individuals interviewed for this book came from diverse backgrounds. They were graduates of the 1940s, 1950s, 1960s, 1970s, and 1980s. All but one were female. The basic nursing education of the registered nurses was at the diploma, associate-degree, and baccalaureate-degree levels. One participant was a licensed practical nurse. The highest degree held was the doctorate; four individuals had law degrees. A few had experiences as nurse educators and some were in that role concurrent with their elected or appointed positions. Just over half were elected public officials; the remainder were appointees. About 25% claimed Republican as their political affiliation; about 60% claimed Democrat; one individual (about 2%) claimed Independent; and the remainder maintained a nonpartisan stance, mainly because their public offices precluded claiming allegiance to one party. One participant who claimed to be nonpartisan said that "You can play politics but cannot get caught."

The clinical specialty background of participants was no less varied. Their backgrounds were in community/public health, emergency room, pediatrics, psychiatric nursing, dialysis, occupational health, critical care, oncology, obstetrics, bone transplant, medical-surgical nursing, and gerontology. Several had experience with national and/or state nurses' organizations, either as students or professionals. Two had been volunteers in the Peace Corps and several had volunteered in their communities on school and hospital boards, parent-teacher associations, and local planning boards, in churches and synagogues, and on political campaigns. These individuals felt that the "training ground" for their current position included these experiences.

Some of those who ran for office were prompted to do so by an extraordinary event in their lives. For example, Lois Capps supported her husband in a congressional race that he won in 1996. Shortly thereafter, they were involved in a car accident with a drunk driver that left her husband unable to fulfill his commitment.

He died suddenly in 1997, and this propelled Capps to run for office. Although she had not before seen the leadership potential in herself, she learned a great deal from campaigning with her husband. During that campaign, she had discussed health and education issues, both of which were high priorities to her. She knew the issues and knew how to run. First elected in 1996, Carolyn McCarthy was motivated to run for office following a shooting spree on a train in December 1993 that left her husband dead and her son critically injured. This personal tragedy became her *raison d'etre* for fighting for gun control. She is a staunch advocate for gun control, including legislation to ban assault weapons. Although not influenced by a single extraordinary event, Judy Robson experienced a number of injustices in her life that she wanted "to right." For example, as a child she felt discriminated against because she couldn't be a batboy. As a young pregnant woman, she had her traineeship taken away because she was told that she was unlikely to work after her schooling. She said that nurses like to be rescuers. As a legislator she "rescues a lot of people"; she advocates for them.

Why do nurses get involved in politics? Nursing and politics have been inseparable since the beginning of the modern nursing movement. Concern for nursing education and practice, as well as politically important questions of the period, such as public health or woman suffrage, interested the politically active nurse at the beginning of the 20th century. Their nursing background taught them the essentials of good citizenship and self-government. While students, they learned about their civic responsibilities and how to participate in government. Nurses who were political activists saw a distinct relationship between their education and social issues of the day. The same moral and social imperative to be a responsible citizen is reflected in the activity of politically minded nurses at the end of the 20th century. Whether they support child labor laws, as they did in the early 1900s, or lobby for the rights of patients in managed care settings in the year 2000, the nurse still must be able to speak to the issues that relate to the health of society. The start of the 21st century gives us pause to look at the role that nurses have played and will continue to play in the public service arena. Nursing professionals have the knowledge and skills that our body politic needs, and have begun to lead the way in determining legislative issues that affect the health of society.

What surfaced during the interviews conducted for this book were a plethora of reasons why these nurses at the turn of the 21st century became involved in politics as candidates and elected and appointed officials. The extension of the nursing role to include policy and politics, "nursing on a grand scale," as one participant said, is totally consistent with nursing's roots in primary health care. In addition to the extraordinary events described above, these nurses' motivations included the desire to serve, a passion for making a difference, an interest in transferring nursing skills to a broader arena, and an inclination for grassroots activism that enables a connection with people.

CREATING THE OPPORTUNITY TO SERVE

When attending a gathering of nurses involved in public policy, Wakefield (1999) observed that:

> The profession has fielded a strong class of individuals who are influencing public policy through an array of positions and activities. Yet, in their conversations they expressed a resounding concern about public policy opportunities ripe for well-prepared nurses but not being pursued. (p. 205)

In her editorial, Wakefield gave suggestions that could be implemented by nursing faculty to develop a "policy work force," for example, educational experiences that go beyond the classroom, faculty role modeling of their own policy activities, coursework that includes policy content, and internships in policy experiences. Armed with a doctorate in public administration and education, Mary Moseley wanted to do something different. She was on a 2-year leave of absence from her tenured faculty position to be with her husband, who was working at the Pentagon during 1996–1997. She thought that if she sent an application to United States Senator Frist (R-Tennessee) it would be "trashed." When she phoned his office to see about a position in the Senator's Washington office, she was told "No." So she decided to just show up. She "dressed right," presented her curriculum vita, and talked her way to a "Yes." Hired by the Senator's Legislative Director, she started out as a fellow, then on staff as an aide to the Senator. Moseley said that when she left, they "didn't want to let me go."

An army nurse for 20 years, Rosemary Nelson "broke the mold" when she seized the opportunity for a leadership position in the area of technology. Having a master's in health care administration, a master's in nursing with a minor in management information systems, and certification in nursing administration and nursing informatics gave her the credentials to develop a computerized patient record for worldwide use by the United States Department of Defense (DOD). The computerized record "moves with the patient," making it possible to track military personnel and veterans throughout the world to provide and monitor care. Through this work Nelson has been recognized and was transferred to the position of Chief Information Officer for the Pacific Rim, where she has been working on telehealth and telemedicine applications, validating commercial and emerging technology, and conducting clinical informatics research. A major accomplishment has been the way nurses are viewed by others in the DOD. She believes that nurses "must groom clinical champions" who can pursue nontraditional roles such as hers.

Susan Reinhard spent a number of years in education and policy activities. She was hired as Director of Policy and Research for the state of New Jersey because the person who hired her was looking for someone who knew research and policy issues and was "based in reality." He wanted someone who had a sense of timing in the political arena. As Policy Director, she spent time looking at policies to enhance the quality of life of seniors in New Jersey. She put forth her ideas to the governor to fold senior services into one department. Governor Christine Todd Whitman accepted her idea and created the Department of Health and Senior Services. Reinhard was appointed Deputy Commissioner of this department in July 1996. In this role, she has been able to implement initiatives she had envisioned since she was a community health nurse. She has been a prime mover on a number of bills, including third-party reimbursement and prescriptive privileges for advanced practice nurses. She has worked to increase the number of dollars available for home and community based care, particularly focusing on ways to keep seniors in their homes during times of illness and disability and to provide respite care for family caregivers.

When she moved to Maryland in 1964, Paula Hollinger was unable to vote in the presidential election that year because of a

1-year residency requirement. So she became a volunteer in the election and got involved in local politics. In 1976 she was a delegate for then Governor Jimmy Carter and did well in vote-getting. In fact, she did such a good job getting votes for others, that she decided that she could probably outdo them! She wanted to run for delegate assembly in Maryland and, with the help of many friends, ran in 1978, 1982, and 1986. In the third election, Hollinger challenged an incumbent and won. She was reelected in 1990. After redistricting in 1994 led to competition with an incumbent (80% of the new district was in the incumbent's district and not hers), she got two-thirds of the vote. In 1985, Hollinger pursued her goal of bringing 3-year nurses "back to the fold." She put forth a bill to have blanket credit for diploma and associate degree nursing graduates in Maryland applied toward baccalaureate degree programs in nursing. Although the bill passed the Maryland House of Representatives, it did not pass in the Senate. Despite this, she was able to create a transition program for 2- and 3-year graduates that allows up to 60 credits transferred through validation. This nationally known model is still in existence in Maryland.

Having taken a nurse refresher course after a long absence from nursing practice, Mary McGrattan had difficulty finding a job. Not long after starting to work in a long- term care facility, "the last thing I wanted to go into," she learned that the man who was the Connecticut State Representative was retiring. She thought, "Ah, I think I would like that job." Since the state legislative position was part-time, she could also continue to work in clinical practice. She ran and won and started her fourth term in 1999. Patricia Montoya said she was in the right place at the right time and was willing to take the risk. By virtue of her being a woman, a nurse, and a Hispanic, opportunities were created as she was sought for political positions. While she had no preset plan for a political career, she had a lot of drive, was not satisfied with the status quo, and wanted to make a difference.

THE INGREDIENT OF PASSION

In 1987 and again in 1998, Meleis addressed the nursing community through her keynote speeches and writings about "a passion for substance." In the first iteration (Meleis, 1987), she identified the visions of the nursing leadership of the past and identified four "reVisions of our visions," namely, a passion for substance, gender-sensitive knowledge, a global approach, and joy and engagement in knowledge development. She also established markers on the reVisions path, saying that "three areas of accountability are signs that we are on the right road: (1) accountability to the domain of nursing; (2) accountability to humanity; and (3) accountability to ourselves" (Meleis, 1987, p. 73). The first reVision, a passion for substance, has great relevance for the nurse in a public position; Meleis is making the point that we must have passion for the business of nursing. In her later writing, a reprint of the original article is accompanied by her "reflections" (1998b). It is entitled, "A Passion for Making a Difference: ReVisions for Empowerment." She adds three new reVisions, the first of which is a passion for making a difference. This passion is directed toward "doing everything we can to make a significant difference in the care of our clients . . . [and] . . . making a difference in the lives of communities that nurses serve" (p. 89). Chinn (cited in Luther, 1995) also recognized the importance of passion when she remarked:

> For the remainder of this century, the most worthy goal that nurses can select is that of arousing their passion for a kind of political activism that will make a difference in their own lives and in the life of our society. (p. 6)

This is no less true as we begin the 21st century. The ingredient of passion is still a prime reason to get involved.

As a child of the 1960s, Virginia Trotter Betts wanted to change the world. She said that nurses change lives every day. She brought the same passion of clinical nursing into the arena of public service. She grew up in a family that tried to make a difference in their community. Her mother was a public health nurse in Appalachia; her father was a postal worker. Her parents led by example, and she attended a nursing school where service was also an expectation. Her most recent impact has been in raising the presence of nursing in the United States Department of Health and Human Services. While health provider has usually meant "physician," Betts has been successfully promoting the concept of health provider as inclusive of nurses and others. A passion for health care issues has also made for the success of

Lois Capps. Those issues include "huge managed care problems," where managed care companies are "pulling out, leaving seniors at home without care."

Robson (1998) said:

> As a young Kennedy idealist [of the 1960s], I heeded his call to government service, which paralleled my attraction to nursing. I viewed both as a special way to meet the needs of the voiceless, the powerless, and the most vulnerable, and to make a difference. (p. 426)

Mel Callan became a nurse practitioner in the 1970s, about the time that then New York Governor Nelson Rockefeller advocated restrictions on nursing legislation for nurse practitioners, having initially vetoed the state's Nurse Practice Act. She became involved in legislative issues because of her passion for this particular issue. She then became active in the New York State Nurses Association and expanded her political activism to include other health-related issues. Christine Canavan was "fed up with the state of health care." She saw her dialysis patients being compromised because of insurance and government regulations. Regulations were not being enforced; there were too many patients to serve at one time, and this was unsafe. While watching C-SPAN one day, she saw a program about women running for office, one of whom was a nurse. The women talked about door-to-door campaigning and the fact that "you don't need to know everything in order to run." Canavan decided to run for the Massachusetts State Legislature and won.

When giving advice about being a political appointee, Shirley Chater said that you "need to be passionate about what you will be doing." She demonstrated this passion when she pushed for reform of the United States Social Security Administration (SSA) to be more customer-focused so that "it works better and costs less." This took persistence and persuasion, because it meant that first the SSA employees would have to work together as a team—something they initially resisted. Susan Reinhard was known as someone who worked in a "passionate way," someone who was passionate about nursing and the services she provided. She wanted to change the system to help people and has succeeded in making a difference for seniors in New Jersey. Nancy

Valentine said, "One must be driven to make a difference." Indeed, she has made a difference on many fronts because of her passion. For example, she was instrumental in expanding the work and number of advanced practice nurses in the Veterans Administration. This has been accomplished by cross-training clinical specialists throughout the country and increasing access to nursing education through the first national distance learning program offered by the Uniform Services University, partnering with universities around the country. She also was effective in increasing the presence of clinical nurse specialists and nurse practitioners in the Veterans Administration.

DEVELOPING POLITICAL SKILLS

Nursing skills are political skills. That was a message heard clearly and often in the interviews of elected and appointed officials. In discussing the fourth stage of nursing's political development, Cohen et al. (1996) describe some of the political skills that are critical to reshaping the health care system, including coalition-building, grassroots mobilization, issue-based collaboration, building a constituency, risk-taking, public media expertise, and background in policy analysis and related research. Cowart (1977) speaks to knowledge of the legislative process, i.e., "how bills are initiated, shaped, amended, and made into law" (p. 777), as an important political skill. As Vice Chair of the Committee on Health Policy of the Tennessee Nurses Association, Summers (1996) wrote that nurses can "make a difference by following the three Cs of Political Influence: Communication, Collectivity, Collegiality" (p. 37). Similarly, Hanley (1987) refers to four modes of political behavior, i.e., voting, campaigning, communal activity, and protest. These skills are coupled with hard facts, information, and research. Backer, Costello-Nikitas, Mason, McBride, and Vance (1993) advanced a feminist model of caring that "encompasses the values of wholeness, interconnectedness, equality, process, support, diversity, and collaboration" (p. 71). They said that these values contrast with "dominant societal values of individualism, competition, and inequality" (p. 71) and are compatible with nurses' values and a new world view that supports the development of skills for "policy formulation and implementation" (p. 69).

One nurse said that people listened to her because she was a nurse and because she came prepared with the facts. In describing how her political skills developed, another nurse said that the major medical center where she worked earlier in her career was a "political institution," which is probably true of many of the sites where nurses practice. Others explained that research from nursing and other disciplines informed the policy decisions that they advocated and made. Mary Wakefield, for example, said that in her position as Director of the Center for Health Policy and Ethics at George Mason University she engages in and analyzes research that affects health and health care policy.

In quoting Marilyn Goldwater, Meyer (1992) wrote:

> "I think all the skills we develop as nurses are transferable to the political arena—the ability to be organized, to listen and be sensitive and perceptive, to communicate with people of all socioeconomic levels, to get things done." To these skills she adds nursing's knowledge of the health-care system and their "compassion and caring." (p. 56)

All of these skills were identified during the interviews. Other skills identified were observing body language, risk-taking behaviors, knowing how to "work the system" vis-a-vis negotiation, the art of debate, knowing when to back off and when to make your case, and having a breadth of interest well beyond nursing and health care. Beth Mazzella said:

> The art of negotiating, of compromise, of knowing when to draw lines in the sand, knowing how to make your presentation, how to build alliances and coalitions—all of those things have to come together for you to survive [as a political appointee].

Eve Franklin believes that "you must know the rules. You must balance altruism with pragmatism to survive and be effective [in politics]." Donna Gentile O'Donnell said, "Going down a river you need to learn to read the water, understand the nuance, to go around the rocks and things hidden just below the surface of the water. You need to learn the technical skill of politics, e.g., people in politics make promises that they don't always keep . . . the nuances of politics." When you are unprepared for high-level politics, as was Kristine Gebbie, the rocks are difficult to avoid. When Gebbie went to The White House as "AIDS Czar," she "underestimated the complexity of the federal system and her ability to make change." She said that there was no apprenticeship and, because of that, she was "working uphill." Her post was created by President Clinton by fiat, without congressional backing, and there was no structure or budget associated with the position. She felt she "lacked D.C. sophistication" that was necessary to develop her department. This was coupled by pressures on the administration to be better organized, affecting her ability to "read the waters." Despite the adversities, she was able to make structural changes that persisted after she left her position.

A question asked of each participant was how he or she developed the political skills needed to carry out their work. Some people referred to their work with student and professional state and national nurses associations. For example, Virginia Trotter Betts was President of the Tennessee State Nurses Association and, subsequently, the American Nurses Association. She also developed her political skills as a Robert Wood Johnson fellow in the late 1980s. Sheila Burke was exposed to nursing organizations through her student nurses' association. She was one of the individuals involved in establishing Nurses for Political Action (NPA) (Rothberg, 1985), New York's forerunner to the national Nurses' Coalition for Action in Politics (N-CAP), currently known as ANA-PAC, the political action arm of the ANA. Mel Callan, past President of the New York State Nurses Association (NYSNA), was encouraged by NYSNA to get involved with local politics. Pat Latona and Margaret Leonard were also active in NYSNA at both state and local levels. Mary Wakefield was involved with the North Dakota Nurses Association prior to 1987 when she moved to Washington. This experience gave way to her interest in legislative initiatives and her subsequent work as a legislative assistant to North Dakota Senator Quentin Burdick. She eventually became the Senator's Chief of Staff.

As a member of the New Jersey State Nurses Association (NJSNA), Susan Reinhard joined the Legislative Committee, learned how a bill became a law, and lobbied part-time. While a faculty member at Rutgers—The State University of New Jersey, she was hired by NJSNA to lobby one day a week. As a lobbyist, she learned to explain, in 2–3 minutes, nursing and the issue she was supporting. She shared this expertise with her students and encouraged them to practice this skill. She took students to Trenton to hear a bill being discussed on the Senate floor. The bill was designed to not allow feeding tubes to be removed regardless of the request of the patient or family. The bill had passed the Assembly and was being considered by the Senate. Reinhard described how her students "grabbed Senators in the lobby of the building and spoke with them about this bill. The students [were effective in changing] the decision . . . the Senators held the bill and stopped its passage." Judy Robson was active in the ANA as Congressional District Coordinator and President of her district nurses' association. These are some of the activities that drew her to politics and, along with her nursing background, prepared her as a problem-solver and team player and to be organized and have "great people skills" and "lots of stamina" (Robson, 1998, p. 432). Muriel Shore was President of NJSNA when Barbara Wright was Executive Director. Wright was at the same time Mayor of Plainsboro, New Jersey. Shore thrived on hearing of Wright's experiences as mayor and Wright encouraged Shore to run for Mayor of Fairfield, New Jersey.

Shirley Chater said that her route to developing political skills was trial and error, observing others, excellent mentors, and friends and colleagues she could trust. Alison Giles credited her family and educational background for her political skills. As a nurse and lawyer, she developed the skills for public service. Growing up in the Washington, DC area, family discussions of politics helped her as well. Eileen Cody's experience in union work helped her to learn the process of negotiating, including when to move and when to withdraw. Paula Hollinger developed political skills through the campaigns of others, by supporting local and national candidates. Once she was sworn in to the Massachusetts State Legislature, Kay Khan joined caucuses, for example, the progressive caucus ("as a Liberal Democrat, it was a good fit") and the women's caucus. She used these opportunities to learn the legislative process and form a network for mutual support of bills. Among her political skills is perseverance. She said, "You need to keep fighting and pushing."

Eve Franklin said that she "finds politics liberating because you don't have to pretend you don't have an agenda. Everyone has an agenda and you are up front about what it is." As someone who is very direct in her interactions with others, Sharon Cooper experienced some difficulty in developing the "backroom" political skills acceptable in southern Georgia. She said that the reason may have been cultural differences, since her students also had trouble with her directness, or it could have been a gender issue since Georgia politics is definitely still male-dominated. Her pro-life stance alienated her from the support of the Georgia Nurses Association. Beverly Nelson-Forbes shared that she is "not much of a politician but what I am is dead honest and a hard worker . . . how I play the political game is tell it like it is and sometimes that'll do it." Christine Canavan said she had to learn "what NOT to say" and confessed that she sometimes has "foot in mouth" syndrome. It is an "ongoing process to develop [political] skills." Still working on her skills, Nancy Valentine said, "You need to learn to have a thick skin . . . there is backbiting and internal jealousies and you need to be political. When they kick you in the stomach, smile and thank them for their support."

SHARING POWER

"Power can be intoxicating. Success is reinforcing, but you need to keep grounded in purpose and direction," so advised Bonnie Ryan. Over 20 years ago, Diers (1978) spoke of the power of numbers in nursing when she said:

> If as nurses we all stopped worrying about all the things that sep-
> arate us from each other—training, degrees, geography, employ-
> ment setting, specialty—and started to worry together about where
> nursing will fit in a reshaped health care system, how much energy
> could we generate? And how much power? For power in numbers
> to be perceived as powerful, the numbers have to be visible in the
> right places. (p. 52)

Even earlier in time, Ashley (1973) spoke of the failure of nurses to recognize and use power effectively. She wrote, "Many nurses . . . seem to feel powerless or feel that the power they do have is unimportant. Now, more than ever before a sense of doom seems to pervade the nursing profession" (p. 637). Indeed, the many opposing forces both within and outside of nursing reinforced the powerlessness of those times. In response, according to Bullough and Bullough (1984) nurses sought power within their own ranks because they were "denied power in the male dominated world" (p. 68). They recognized that although nursing had developed power, it "was concentrated on the internal world of nursing" (p. 68). As a political force, nurses have come a long way. Take the example of Sheila Burke, as reflected in the writings of DeParle (1995): "Day to day, Burke does more to shape the [United States] Senate's agenda than all but a handful of its actual members" (p. 34). Overall, individual nurses and organized nursing have been instrumental during the past decade in shaping public policy and health policy objectives at all levels of government and the public sector. Yet there is so much more to be done.

Mason (1999) refers to the political skill of sharing power "in ways that respect and value differences. It's how to develop and use a process of consensus building" (p. 7). Mason, Backer, and Georges (1991) also include sharing power in describing a feminist model of empowerment, i.e., "respect for others and for self, power-sharing, and equality" (p. 73). Terry (1993) calls this empowering leadership a "power-with perspective," noting that it "lies at the heart of efforts by political or social movements, community organizers, and citizen renewal projects to mobilize people to define and secure their own agendas" (p. 33). While the notion of empowerment is not new, it has been recast in the feminist view in an effort to create strength in the political skills of nurses. Two articles (Mason et al., 1991; Sohier, 1992) address ways in which nurses can develop and use power based on the notion of empowerment. In the first, Mason et al. describe the potential power of nurses and the need to increase political awareness and skills. They define empowerment as "the enabling of individuals and groups to participate in actions and decision-making within a context that supports an equitable distribution of power" (pp. 72–73).

When describing their impact on political processes and outcomes, several participants indicated how they shared power and used the process of consensus building to address issues. Power sharing came in the form of co-sponsoring bills, being involved in women's caucuses to deal with common issues, agreeing to serve on legislative committees, working with state and national nursing organizations to advance policies, and what Kay

Khan refers to as "forming, developing, and keeping relation-ships." Cindy Empson says that "it's difficult to claim having an impact as an individual. It takes a lot of people working togeth-er." Beth Mazzella described the Federal Nursing Service Council as a support group that became a "proactive group trying to advance nursing and health agendas in the federal sector" and represents the ideals of respect, equality, and power sharing. The group is composed of women in charge of the various Nurse Corps, that is, the Chief Nurse of the Army, Navy, Air Force, Veterans Administration, Public Health Service and the American Red Cross.

In an effort to "bring federal and state government closer to the people of Marshalltown," Beverly Nelson-Forbes has led sum-mits to Washington, DC, and Des Moines, Iowa. She felt that the approximately 27,000 people of Marshalltown never really paid attention to the political process, nor had they been empowered to do so. The summits provide an opportunity to "work the process," to "not just sit back and complain about what the state is doing or not doing, but making an effort to have their voices heard." This is an excellent example of empowerment in that it fosters development of consciousness about issues and the polit-ical skills needed to affect change. According to Hall-Long (1995), this kind of collaboration with the public not only helps to "pro-mote the nation's health . . . [but also promotes] . . . the public policy-making role of the nursing profession" (p. 28). Another example is the view of Herschella Horton that "what counts is not the number of bills, but being able to help others to have access to health care, to empower others." She educates people in her community in health care matters, especially economic develop-ment, and talks to them about the political process, that is, "how to impact it and make your voice heard . . . I try to teach people how to be effective."

On her first month or two on the job, her employees "sized up" Shirley Chater. Their attitude was that she was temporary. She kept pushing the agenda that their opinions mattered and that they would work together as a group. She discussed the antici-pated positive impact of this approach on the agency. Although it took time and persistence, the message eventually became clear that they were a team. This approach is certainly support-ive of what Mason and Leavitt (1995) say about political power:

"The individual activist is needed to provide the vision and role modeling, but the greatest potential lies with the collective" (p. 46).

In the second article that focused on the notion of empowerment, Sohier (1992) said:

We must empower each other by recognizing and centering on the incipient potency of nursing knowledge . . . our first task is to raise the consciousness of nurses by describing the fundamental power contained in nursing knowledge and by doing so from "womanist" perspectives. (p. 62)

Well accepted is the fact that knowledge is power. "Knowledge empowers," says Meleis (1998a, p. 93). When referring to the many accomplishments of the nursing profession in advancing nursing knowledge, she further states: "We can no longer afford to develop knowledge that does not influence health care policies" (p. 94).

According to Leonhardt (1998), nurses have been successful as a political force by:

1. becoming familiar with the types of issues in debate;
2. taking into account the various environments where health care issues matter;
3. identifying the arenas where nursing's political clout can be best utilized to accomplish change;
4. evaluating the stakeholders; and
5. recognizing the resources available, both financial and human, to win nursing's issues. (p. 14)

Having this kind of knowledge is potentially very powerful. Knowledge as empowerment was clearly voiced by Kate Malliarakis, who said that her nurse practitioner training was "a real turning point for me to look 'beyond the box' . . . [it] empowered me with knowledge about myself."

EXPANDING ONE'S KNOWLEDGE BASE

While it is absolutely essential to develop and use nursing knowledge in the way Meleis (1998a) advocates, the policymaker who is a nurse must go well beyond this frame of reference. Concern was voiced by some of the nurses interviewed that while their nursing education facilitated their work in office, they needed to expand their scope of interest and knowledge. To fully serve in the public arena, nurses needed to understand the implications of health care as they relate to other issues in society. Nurses must broaden their horizons and be globally aware. When coupled with their nursing background, reading the paper, keeping up on current events, and acknowledging other disciplines has produced unique and successful public servants.

Mary Wakefield said that nurses cannot be speaking just "nurse speak." Having breadth in topics she could discuss with people "really provided an entrée, whether I was meeting the Governor of the State or the representative of General Electric . . . or someone in transportation where I could talk about the latest Amtrak activity." Wakefield noted that you must engage individuals on their turf about their interests, and let them see that you are paying attention to the issues. Marilyn Lee is supportive of the idea that nurses must look outward, not inward. She said that nurses need to know what is going on in their communities and to interact with others to learn about the issues. When she was elected to her community advisory board, she became involved in zoning issues and roads, topics far from the insular focus of many nurses. When giving advice to anyone who may be interested in a policy role, Allison Giles said, "be active in causes, be broad thinking beyond the individual patient."

Patricia Montoya wanted to broaden her background to be able to speak to issues beyond child health, so she sought positions in home health and managed care and got master's degrees in public administration and health administration. She felt that these credentials gave her a broader perspective on the health care system and a higher degree of understanding of Medicaid, managed care, and third party reimbursement. She knew how the system worked and this added to her credibility with legislators and the public. Carolyn McCarthy confessed that she knew nothing when she ran for Congress. She went on her "gut feelings," doing what she thought was right. She said that nurses see things as a whole, i.e., holistically, and that you can't legislate without looking at the broader picture. She gave the following example: "As a nurse caring for a cardiac patient, you know that it affects the whole family so you include the family in your plan of care. The same goes for legislation."

FOSTERING CONNECTIONS THROUGH GRASSROOTS ACTIVISM

In writing about nursing and politics in the United States, Smith (1991) described Lavinia Dock's crusade for equal rights: "She marched in Washington and went to jail for her belief in equal rights for women" (p. 7). Dock also used the power of the pen to promote activism on behalf of women to oppose discriminatory labor laws and to support the Equal Rights Amendment (Reverby, 1985). Her editorials appeared in nursing journals and attempted to inform nurses and propel them to action. Martha Minerva Franklin "worked for collective action by Black nurses in the early twentieth century" (Bullough, Church, & Stein, 1988). Because Black nurses were excluded from membership in state nurses associations and, consequently, from the ANA, her intent was to start an organization where their voices could be heard. Between 1906 and 1907, Franklin mailed 1,500 letters to Black nurses who had attended historically Black schools of nursing to ascertain their concerns. Out of this grew the National Association of Colored Graduate Nurses (NACGN).

Margaret Sanger is a third example of the early political activists in nursing who used grassroots activism to support their causes. Sanger started a newspaper, *Woman Rebel,* to begin a dialogue about the right of women "to choose whether or not to have children" (Lewenson, 1998, p. 52). She also published on syphilis in a socialist newspaper, *The Call,* but the "issue was declared unmailable because of the nature of the material . . ." (Lewenson, p. 52). Her crusade for choice brought her from New York City to Europe, where she sought out safe contraception measures. After returning to New York in 1916, "Sanger, along with her sister, opened the first birth control clinic in the Brownsville section of Brooklyn" (Lewenson, p. 52). On more than one occasion she faced arrest, prosecution, and imprisonment, but she persevered. These examples of grassroots activism laid the path for the nurses of today who have used this strategy to connect with people, hear their concerns, and be effective in representing their interests. Nursing is in an ideal position to make changes at the grassroots level because of the trust the public places in nurses.

Terry (1993) wrote, "Grassroots people are authentic" (p. 33). Grassroots activism is one way for elected and appointed officials to connect with their constituents, colleagues, and organizations within their communities. Lobbying is not reserved for professional lobbyists. Citizens lobby, lawmakers lobby, and small and large organizations lobby. Robson (1998) discusses three keys to effective grassroots lobbying, preparation, politeness, and perseverance. Legislators need votes and they need support. As a lobbyist Susan Reinhard had to get in, make the point, and close in 2–3 minutes. She had to explain nursing and the issue during this time frame. Quite a challenge, but obviously effective, based on her track record! Janegale Boyd had her first lobbying experience as a volunteer with the American Lung Association. Mary Moseley said:

> It's never too late to be schooled in grassroots lobbying. You need to target the right groups working on specific legislation. You need to know how bills become laws. You need to have data to support what you say. You need to keep in constant contact with legislators to be effective.

For nurse candidates and elected officials, grassroots activism played a critical role when they campaigned for office and in their day-to-day work. It provided a way to be in touch with community values and concerns. For example, Paula Hollinger's campaign literature said "This nurse makes house calls." She has attended many community functions, did a local newspaper column, and generally goes out a lot in her neighborhood and sees people that way. She said that her grocery store is her "district office." She feels that contacting your state legislator on issues has a tremendous impact. Eddie Bernice Johnson spends a lot of her time touring plants and hospitals to "get a real feel for what is going on." In the state of Iowa they have a citizens legislature, reports Beverly Nelson-Forbes.

> We are there from January to April; a hundred days one year and 110 days the second year . . . they want you to have another job. They don't want full-time legislators. They want people who have a job who are out in the public to see what the working day world is like . . .
>
> They want you to be a part of the community, work in the community, then come to the legislature with a better idea of what the needs of the community are.

Kay Khan uses a variety of strategies to reach out to her constituents and involve them in the political process. For example, she works with individuals; meets with groups who need something done in their community, such as environmental and transportation issues; holds office hours for constituents to meet with her; and uses cable television to reach out and bring issues to her constituents. A newer way to connect with constituents is through the Internet. So says Marilyn Lee, who started her own website so she could communicate with the people in her district. She also started a caregivers' support group to reach out to constituents. She has an open door, believing what former Speaker of the House of Representatives Tip O'Neill is often quoted as having said: "All politics is local."

Mary McGrattan said that 50% of her time is spent helping people. People call her with individual problems, "problems with motor vehicles, divorce, you name it. You try to direct them to the right person or make a phone call on their behalf. They're so pleased, so thankful because they just weren't able to do it." Having led eight summits to Washington, DC, Beverly Nelson-Forbes engages her community to make their voices heard, both at the state level and federally. She learned several things from these experiences. First, she learned that the constituents who got together to go to the summits didn't know each other, much less their elected officials. Second, she learned that the people she met at the state and federal levels were "human." So she had the firsthand opportunity to learn the issues from her constituents and meet some of the people who could address these issues with her. Maureen O'Connell feels that her job is to be in touch with the people that she represents, "to hear their everyday problems and concerns." People don't usually ask her what bill she voted for; instead, they want to know about the issues that are of concern to them, given the circumstances of their lives, "whether it's taxes on small business, or crime issues in the community, or juvenile delinquency, or health concerns."

His work in the health care field put Joseph Polisena in touch with "the average Jane or Joe." He was elected following a grass-roots door-to-door campaign where he focused on issues not being addressed. He feels it is important to be in contact with people, even if he is unable to help them. Mary Simmons "walked the entire city" when she campaigned for office. She asked people their concerns and didn't make any promises. Wherever she goes to speak, she tells people that she can take constructive criticism. She says:

> If you disagree with me, certainly call and let me know. If you have an idea, my best ideas come from my constituents. Let me know because I can't think of everything. Something may not be working for you that I have no clue about because I'm not involved in it, like maybe elder health insurance or something else.

GETTING THE JOB DONE

Throughout grassroots interactions, public support has had a significant positive impact throughout the country. The following examples illustrate these positive outcomes:

• During review of health laws under the Alcohol and Drug Law in Pennsylvania, it was determined that the state's legal age of adulthood of 14 prevented parents from intervening to get treatment for their children who used drugs. As a result of this review, Patricia Vance was prime sponsor on legislation to change the legal age from 14 to 18. The legislation passed the House twice but was stalled in the Senate. A woman who had been in touch with Vance knew that her son was in desperate trouble, but she was helpless to intercede. The suicide of her 14-year-old son propelled this mother to move Vance's cause forward. She visited every senator until the bill was enacted.

• In the Borough of Queens in New York City, Claire Shulman is trying "to make sure health care is available to everybody, accessible to everybody regardless of ethnicity, race, or ability to pay." This is a borough with "170 languages and dialects . . . [and] . . . the largest immigrant population in New York City." She is acutely aware of the health needs of her community because she is a nurse. "I don't think anyone sitting in my chair who is not a nurse would engage in this. It happens to be because I'm a nurse that I'm interested in this subject." So she makes a sincere effort to get the job done. She has a person on staff who is overseeing immunization and a retired nurse has offered to do immunizations pro bono. There are mobile units that go from neighborhood to neighborhood giving the appropriate immunizations. She has health fairs in community neighborhoods where medical services are less available, and a pulmonary and asthma mobile van that goes to areas where there is a high population of children with asthma.

• Muriel Shore developed several programs for seniors in Fairfield, New Jersey, including a Senior Resource Center equipped a room with technology for seniors to learn computer skills and a recreational program for seniors (LIFES) that addresses health needs and activities of daily living. She has worked to "move the focus of government to environmental and quality of life issues" because she cares about people and is committed to moving nursing's agenda forward.

• By bringing women and their babies to the House of Representatives, Eileen Cody was able to demonstrate the effectiveness of involving the community in a grassroots effort to "enable 'family-friendly' businesses to encourage breast feeding." The women breastfed their infants during the legislative session. While the legislation passed in the House, the Senate defeated the bill. She will introduce it again this year and thinks it will pass ("They're tired of listening to me about this").

• Working with the nursing community, Barbara Wright sponsored legislation for nurses to have prescriptive authority for controlled substances for terminally ill patients. Ideally, she wanted the authority to extend to all patients, but compromise was necessary to get the bill through. The legislation allows nurses to prescribe controlled substances for terminally ill patients and renew and adjust prescriptions for controlled substances for patients who are not terminally ill.

• Another important bill that had a great deal of community support and a national audience was Megan's Law. This "significant, influential piece of legislation" focused on victim's rights. Megan was a child who was raped and murdered by a known sex offender. She lived in Wright's district. The bill calls for community notification when a known sex offender is residing in the community. This law was quite controversial, as laws are generally designed to protect the rights of the accused; implementation has been controversial as well, both within New Jersey and around the country.

There are many more examples of the responsiveness of nurses
to community issues that involve the mobilization of community resources. Their stories are impressive and often powerful. The next chapter provides additional exemplars of the way
nurses address social issues and impact on political processes
and outcomes.

REFERENCES

Ashley, J. A. (1973). About power in nursing. *Nursing Outlook, 21*(10),
    637–641.
Backer, B. A., Costello-Nikitas, D., Mason, D. J., McBride, A. B., &
    Vance, C. (1993). Power at the policy table: When women and
    nurses are involved. *Revolution: The Journal of Nurse Empower-
    ment, 3,* 68–76.
Bullough, V. L., & Bullough, B. (1984). Nurses and power: Professional
    power vs. political clout. *Women & Politics, 4*(4), 67–75.
Bullough, V. L., Church, O. M., & Stein, A. P. (1988). *American nursing: A
    biographical dictionary.* New York: Garland.
Clayton, S. L. (1993). Address of S. Lillian Clayton. In N. Birnbach & S. B.
    Lewenson (Eds.), *Legacy of Leadership: Presidential addresses from
    the Superintendents' Society and the National League of Nursing Edu-
    cation 1894–1952* (pp. 138–143). New York: National League for
    Nursing Press. (Original work published 1919)
Cohen, S. S., Mason, D. J., Kovner, C., Leavitt, J. K., Pulcini, J., &
    Sochalski, J. (1996). Stages of nursing's political development:
    Where we've been and where we ought to go. *Nursing Outlook, 44,*
    259–265.
Cowart, M. E. (1977). Teaching the legislative process. *Nursing Outlook,
    25,* 777–780.
DeParle, J. (1995, November 12). Sheila Burke is the militant feminist
    commie peacenik who's telling Bob Dole what to think. *The New
    York Times Magazine,* pp. 32–38, 90, 100, 102–104.
Diers, D. (1978). A different kind of energy: Nurse power. *Nursing
    Outlook, 26,* 51–55.
Findings from the national sample survey of registered nurses—March
    1996. (1997). United States Department of Health and Human Services
    Health Resources and Services Administration Bureau of Health
    Professions Division of Nursing.
Hall-Long, B. A. (1995). Nursing's past, present, and future political
    experiences. *Nursing & Health Care, 16,* 24–28.

Hanley, B. E. (1987, July/August). Political participation: How do nurses compare with other professional women? *Nursing Economic$, 5*(4), 179–185.

Leonhardt, M. A. (1998). Nursing as a political force. *Connecticut Nursing News, 71*(1), 14.

Lewenson, S. B. (1998). Historical overview: Policy, politics, and nursing. In D. J. Mason & J. K. Leavitt (Eds.), *Policy and politics in nursing and health care* (3rd ed., pp. 41–58). Philadelphia: Saunders.

Luther, A. P. (1995). Becoming a more politically active nurse. *ORL— Head and Neck Nursing, 13*(4), 6–10.

Mason, D. J. (1999). Nurses dancing with wolves. *American Journal of Nursing, 99,* 7.

Mason, D. J., Backer, B. A., & Georges, C. A. (1991). Toward a feminist model for the political empowerment of nurses. *Image: Journal of Nursing Scholarship, 23*(2), 72–77.

Mason, D. J., & Leavitt, J. K. (1995). Political activism: The individual versus the collective. *Journal of the New York State Nurses Association, 26,* 46–47.

Meleis, A. (1987). ReVisions in knowledge development: A passion for substance. *Scholarly Inquiry for Nursing Practice, 1*(1), 5–19.

Meleis, A. (1998a). Reflections. A passion for making a difference: ReVisions for empowerment. *Scholarly Inquiry for Nursing Practice, 12*(1), 87–94.

Meleis, A. (1998b). ReVisions in knowledge development: A passion for substance. *Scholarly Inquiry for Nursing Practice, 12*(1), 65–77.

Meyer, C. (1992, October). Nursing on the political front. *American Journal of Nursing, 92,* 56–64.

Reverby, S. (1985). *The history of American nursing: A Lavinia Dock reader.* New York: Garland.

Robson, J. B. (1998). One nurse's journey to becoming a policymaker. In D. Mason & J. K. Leavitt (Eds.), *Policy and politics in nursing and health care* (3rd ed.). Philadelphia: W. B. Saunders.

Rothberg, J. S. (1985). The growth of political action in nursing. *Nursing Outlook, 33*(3), 133–135.

Smith, L. S. (1991). The history of nursing and politics in the United States. *Advancing Clinical Care, 6*(4), 6–7.

Sohier, R. (1992). Feminism and nursing knowledge: The power of the weak. *Nursing Outlook, 35*(1), 62–66, 93.

Summers, B. J. (1996). Nurses and politics: What can we gain? *Tennessee Nurse, 59*(5), 36–37.

Terry, R. W. (1993). *Authentic leadership: Courage in action.* San Francisco: Jossey-Bass.

Wakefield, M. (1999). Public policy: Canaries in the mine. *Journal of Professional Nursing, 15,* 205.

Winter, M. K., & Lockhart, J. S. (1997). From motivation to action: Understanding nurses' political involvement. *Nursing & Health Care Perspectives, 18,* 244–247.

Nurses' Action on Social Issues

> We must take our place in the arena of the world's activities and assume our share of responsibility, endeavoring to work with intelligence and an exalted purpose.
>
> —Lystra Gretter

THE NURSE AS A SOCIAL FORCE

Over time nurses have been involved in social change, being focused on the growth of the profession and the health of society. Nurses have long had a contract with the public to advocate and to "assist the individual, sick or well, in the performance of those activities contributing to health or recovery (or to peaceful death) that he would perform unaided if he had the necessary strength, will or knowledge" (Henderson, 1960, p. 4). Nurses have had a social responsibility to provide care for individuals, families, and groups. Health and politics have been immeasurably intertwined. Through elected and appointed positions, we can continue the tradition and more significantly impact social change, shaping the agenda and leading the way.

As a social force, nursing has early roots. In 1841, prior to the modern nursing movement, Dorothea Dix led a crusade for prisoners who were insane. Traveling from state to state, she advocated

> the creation of state hospitals supported by taxation. Her first victory was in New Jersey in 1845. Taking her concern to the national level, Dix persuaded both houses of Congress to endow institutions for helpless people such as the insane and the blind. (Glass, 1984, p. 40)

Later, following the opening of nurse training schools, Lavinia Dock pursued social reform around such issues as suffrage and venereal disease. Dock's colleague and friend, Lillian Wald, supported social welfare reform, using "the political arena to create change. Her suggestions to the government over a seven-year period ultimately resulted in the establishment of the United States Children's Bureau" (Glass, 1984, p. 39). The modern era of nursing itself began in times of social turbulence and reform. In the late 19th century, the structure of society was changing dramatically, including:

> the role of women, the function of the extended family, educational opportunities, and increasing prosperity. For Nightingale, introducing a new workforce comprising middle class women who hitherto had not been expected to have a role outside the home was a considerable challenge. (Kitson, 1997, p. 112)

Labelle (1986) has identified a number of major issues that affect health, including environmental and social welfare problems, poverty, education, family planning, and population growth. The existence of overcrowded cities, for example, has numerous implications in terms of the economy, energy, and the environment. Food supplies and clean water are two services directly affected by overcrowding. In addition, unemployment may be higher, resulting in more people experiencing poverty. Poverty can lead to malnutrition, which can shorten life expectancy. As well, "chronic infections and anaemia caused by malnutrition . . . saps energy . . . affecting productivity and quality of life" (Labelle, 1986, p. 248). Nursing is concerned with all of these issues, as all are contributing factors to maintaining health. Labelle believes that "by using their levers of power, together with technology and communications, nurses can help create a new world health order" (p. 247).

EXAMPLES OF SOCIAL REFORM BY CONTEMPORARY ORGANIZED NURSING

Built on our history of social reform, we have moved forward to a time and generation where organized nursing has become a social force. Using political action, changes have been brought about on many fronts. Two significant efforts of organized nursing have been in the area of third-party reimbursement and the establishment of the National Institute for Nursing Research (NINR). The first of these reforms was designed to increase access to health care; the second, to improve nursing and health care through research.

Malone and Keepnews (1998) attribute the success of passage of the 1997 bill on Medicare Part B reimbursement for advanced practice registered nurses to "unity, grassroots activism, and most of all, persistence" (p. 298). The nursing community rallied around this legislation, which became effective January 1, 1998, as part of the federal Balanced Budget Act. The path to this social change was not easy, and it came in stages, first with people in nursing homes (1989), then with people in rural areas (1990), and finally in all areas of patient care (1998). This legislation means that there are additional responsibilities for clinical nurse specialists and nurse practitioners about the "broader issues surrounding reimbursement," for example, fraud, abuse, Medicare fee schedules, and appropriate coding of procedures and services. Malone and Keepnews assert that "the biggest challenge nursing now faces is to demonstrate what NPs [nurse practitioners] and CNSs [clinical nurse specialists] really can do for their patients, now that Medicare beneficiaries have access to their services" (p. 300). Amid these successes is a still significant struggle to get reimbursement from private insurers, as documented by Mason, Cohen, O'Donnell, Baxter, and Chase (1997). Managed care organizations were the focal point for their research. They learned that private insurers from the provider panels of approved practitioners overwhelmingly excluded advanced practice registered nurses. The challenge of reform is before us, and organized nursing continues to press on.

The second instance of social reform concerns the efforts of organized nursing to establish an institute within the National Institutes of Health that would focus on nursing research. In 1983, Dr. Ada Sue Hinshaw received a phone call from Congressman Edward Madigan (R-Illinois) to "introduce legislation calling for an institute for nursing research within the National Institutes of Health (NIH)" (Meyer, 1992, p. 59). The Congressman's move in this direction came from an Institute of Medicine report that recommended this support for nursing research. The American Nurses Association met with the other Tri-Council members the National League for Nursing and American Association of Colleges of Nursing (the American Organization of Nurse Executives joined the Tri-Council a few years later), and other nursing leaders to identify the issues and to strategize about the language of such a proposal. The bill was introduced in the fall of 1984 and passed the House of Representatives in November 1984. Nursing leaders then testified in the Senate about "the need to provide a focal point for promoting nursing research and to increase funding for it" (Meyer, 1992, p. 59). In addition, there was a great deal of lobbying behind the scenes.

One of the controversies within the nursing community related to the status of the Division of Nursing once a special research institute would be in place, mainly in relation to funding. There was concern that the funding would be split between the two entities, the proposed institute and the Division of Nursing, and that the Division would lose funding. Because of this concern "nursing leaders struck an agreement to continue support for the Division of Nursing, for education and other programs, helping ease some doubts" (Meyer, 1992, p. 59). Once the Senate and House agreed upon the language of the bill, it was sent to President Reagan for approval. The President vetoed the bill initially, but after further rewriting and compromise, it was approved in 1985 as a "center" rather than a full-fledged institute. It took a total, organized effort to get the foot of nursing in the door of NIH. Again through the legislative efforts of organized nursing, in particular the American Association of Colleges of Nursing, the goal of being named an institute was realized in 1993. The struggle, however, continues in terms of assuring adequate funding to support the many nurse scientists conducting research (only 19% of approved applications are funded, versus 33% of National Institute of Health applications) (Deets, 1999). According to Deets, "more than 20 nursing organizations currently are working to increase NINR's funding. Almost weekly others are joining in the effort to influence senators and representatives to increase the NINR budget to $90.253 million for the year 2000" (p. 80). As it turned out, about $89.5 million has been funded. Requests upward of $110 million have been made for FY2001, with President Clinton recommending $92.5 million (FY2001 President's Budget Press Briefing).

MAJOR ISSUES BROUGHT TO THE TABLE

Although we have just begun to "scratch the surface" in terms of the needs of the public, social reform by individual nurses in public positions has been dramatic. Ample evidence of this impact was provided during the interviews. Major issues that surfaced clustered around a number of areas. These were categorized as follows: tobacco, mental health, seniors, children, women's issues, AIDS, nursing practice, insurance reform, health reform, and other pressing social issues (all others that did not fit into a cluster). The issues within these categories represent contemporary and critical areas for social reform, and are significant challenges to society. To address these areas participants have taken an active role in getting to the table and moving forward the agenda. Their stories are presented here.

USING GAINS FROM TOBACCO CONTROL INITIATIVES

Tobacco presents one excellent example of a health-related issue that has screamed out for social reform. Litigation and legislation in the late 1990s led to the development of individual state tobacco control initiatives, arising from situations where "communities have voiced their needs and preferences and generated pressure on politicians to respond by providing resources" (Atwood, Colditz, & Kawachi, 1997, p. 1604). Through political will, defined as "society's desire and commitment to develop and fund new programs or to modify existing programs" (Atwood et al., 1997, p. 1604), funds have been created for major tobacco control initiatives.

Some of the officials interviewed for this book addressed issues surrounding tobacco control. For example, Kay Khan sponsored a bill in Massachusetts to eliminate smoking advertisements near schools. Although the bill did not pass the first time, she had plans to reintroduce the bill. Also in Massachusetts, Mary Simmons wants to use the money from a tobacco settlement plus the cigar tax to fund placement of a school nurse in every school in the State. Judy Robson is working to ensure that the large tobacco settlement that Wisconsin received will go to anti-smoking measures to discourage children from smoking. In a column addressed to registered nurses, Capps (1998) wrote:

[W]e know that tobacco is extremely addictive and causes an abundance of health problems. We also know that people who don't start smoking in their teen years are much less likely to start at all. We must discourage kids from starting on the road to addiction . . . We can do this by raising the price of cigarettes, ending the glamorization of smoking, and keeping tobacco companies from targeting teens in their ads . . . to pass tobacco legislation we must hear from you. (p. 80)

In discussing issues of importance to Mary McGrattan, she identified an interest in helping the "working poor." These are people who work more than one job but whose companies don't provide health insurance, and these employees can't afford to purchase it themselves. They are not eligible for Medicaid either. She said that in 2000 states like Connecticut are going to receive approximately $44,000,000 from tobacco settlements. She would like to use this money to help the working poor. There may be "some way of subsidizing their employers so that they could get basic medical coverage, so they don't end up in emergency rooms."

ADDRESSING MENTAL HEALTH

While mental illness has been a much avoided topic throughout history, a number of wives of U.S. presidents of the late 20th century have taken up the cause of mental health reform, including mental illness, alcoholism, and drug abuse. Of the nurses interviewed, Herschella Horton, Eve Franklin, Kate Malliarakis, Paula Hollinger, and Kay Khan principally focused on mental health issues, from bills for mental health insurance to employment assistance treatment counseling, to writing "rules" for drug testing, to attempts to get parity between mental health and physical illness treatments, to a Bill of Rights for the mentally ill. They have fought locally, at the state level, and nationally to raise awareness of the public and legislatures about the need to support mental health.

Mental health insurance is a cause that nurses continue to advance. The idea of equal treatment of mental illness and physical illness by insurance companies is more and more gaining voice through the nursing leadership. Legislation on parity has been "difficult to move," said Khan. She has been trying to educate the Massachusetts State Legislature on this by presenting forums with experts and consumers. She is persistent, and said, "You need to keep fighting, pushing." Franklin, too, has been working on a parity bill in Montana for mental health diagnoses, as has Horton in Arizona.

SUPPORTING SENIORS

Because of so many advancements designed to maintain health and prevent and treat illness, people are living longer, and the population of older adults in America has grown geometrically. Wallace, McGuire, Lee, and Sauter (1999) note that "As society ages, the health care system will be faced with increasing numbers of persons with chronic and disabling conditions who have needs for culturally appropriate care" (p. 183). Wallace et al. go on to discuss Healthy People 2000 objectives for elders and how these objectives fit with the provisions of the Older Americans Act of 1995, being considered for reauthorization in the year 2000. Included in the Act are services for seniors, such as home care, health education, disease prevention and promotion services, elder rights and legal assistance programs, multigenerational activities, neighborhood senior care programs, and congregate meals.

The issue of prescription drug costs is of great concern to seniors. In 1992, Wakefield (Mary Wakefield, personal communication, 1992) identified prescription drug costs as one of the most pressing health care concerns facing the country. "Drug prices run about three times the rate of general inflation—and are continuing to skyrocket. The elderly particularly are being hurt by this problem" (Mary Wakefield, personal communication, 1992). Seven years later, in 1999, Carolyn McCarthy took this issue to the United States House of Representatives. McCarthy requested that the House Committee on Government Reform conduct a study concerning prices within her Fourth Congressional District in Nassau County. The prices of five drugs were reviewed in independent and chain stores. Study findings were that "consumers who pay for their own drugs pay more than twice as much for the five monitored medicines as do H.M.O.'s and large insurance companies" (Saslow, 1999, p. 1). This price discrimination has far-reaching implications for the public, particularly for seniors, who often don't have medical insurance. According to the Saslow article:

98 percent of her [McCarthy's] over-65 constituents are on Medicare, which until recently provided benefits that included prescription drugs and small co-payments. But this year, many managed-care plans withdrew their Medicare programs, leaving thousands of elderly Long Islanders without insurance and forced to pay for their prescription drugs out of pocket. (p. 1)

Often, seniors take multiple prescription drugs, and the costs can be impossible to pay. This leads to trade-offs that can gross-ly affect one's health, for example, buying less food (or in some instances eating cat food!) to be able to have money for pre-scription drugs, stopping medications entirely, or selecting some prescriptions to refill and not others. The bill that McCarthy is proposing, the federal Prescription Drug Fairness for Seniors Act of 1999, "would require drug companies to sell to pharmacies that serve Medicare beneficiaries at the same prices as those available to H.M.O.'s and large insurance companies" (Saslow, 1999, p. 15). As of late February 2000, there was no movement on this bill, as it was still in committee. Both Republicans and Democrats, as well as the President, had proposed different bills that address this issue, making the bill very controversial politi-cally (personal conversation with aide to Representative McCarthy, February 23, 2000). On a more local front New Jersey Assemblywoman Barbara Wright has been addressing this issue. Wright has been instrumental in working out an acceptable solu-tion with pharmaceutical companies in New Jersey, where this industry is quite strong. The pharmaceutical industry annually gives $40,000,000 in indigent aid to people who need prescrip-tion drugs.

Mary Simmons, Susan Reinhard, Shirley Chater, Muriel Shore, and Lois Capps have also made the health and welfare of senior citizens a focal point of their work in the public arena. Initiatives have included nutritional programs, special services designed to maintain seniors in their homes, respite care for family caregivers, a Social Security system that is more user-friendly, recreational and educational programs, and trying to ensure that managed care companies support seniors' ability to receive care at home. While at the Social Security Administration, Chater persuaded staff that the agency must be customer-focused. She spoke with consumers, as well, to influence the decisions she made. Reinhard has been effective at the state level in creating an atmosphere that supports the "independence, dignity, and choice" of seniors. She has been effective in getting additional funding in New Jersey for home- and community-based care for seniors and developing a one-stop-shopping system for seniors at the local level to find these services.

ADVOCATING HEALTHY CHILDREN

There is a stanza apropos of advocating healthy children in a poem entitled "The Invitation," written by Oriah Mountain Dreamer, Native American Elder. It reads:

> It doesn't interest me to know where you live or how much money you have. I want to know if you can get up after a night of grief and despair, weary and bruised to the bone, and do what needs to be done for the children.

Herschella Horton read this poem in her keynote address at the 1999 Annual American Holistic Nursing Association conference. It is well known that across the globe millions of children are not being immunized. Although the United States is among the most progressive countries in terms of health care, its immunization statistics are grim. Children who are uninsured or underinsured are, perhaps, the most affected victims. They are also the most vulnerable to a host of illnesses due to malnutrition, poor living conditions, and the like. As referred to in chapter 3, Claire Shulman has made a Herculean effort to ensure that the many uninsured children in Queens, New York are immunized against basic contagious childhood illnesses. She said:

> Besides building roads and sewers, we have been on a campaign to immunize all the children within the borough, because we have so many children from all the countries. We have the largest immigrant population in this city. It's a problem, but we have mobile units that come out, and we go from neighborhood to neighborhood giving them shots.

Judy Robson, Christine Canavan, Barbara Wright, Patricia Vance, and Lois Capps have also attempted to make the lives of children better. They have done so by advocating health care for children and poor families, funding for physically handicapped children, a welfare-to-work program that does not harm children, hearing testing for babies, provision of a school nurse in every school, providing immunization and asthma testing for children, protection for children by changing the legal age of adulthood, and addressing school violence and drug and school safety programs in schools. In 1998, Canavan became aware of the fact that babies in the state of Massachusetts were not tested for hearing loss. She sponsored a bill addressing this that was signed into law in 1999. Wright believes she should be a role model for children and visits fourth grade classes in her district. She tells them what she does, about the public policy role of women, and that she is a nurse. Capps (1998) has taken the lead in Congress "to urge funding for a new Safe and Drug-Free Schools Coordinator Initiative. This program would help recruit, train, and hire counselors for drug and school safety programs in schools" (p. 80). She has also supported legislation on gun control, the Children's Gun Violence Prevention Act of 1998, prohibiting "children from having access to handguns and making parents responsible for keeping loaded firearms out of their reach. Most important, this bill would encourage local gun violence prevention and educational programs for children" (Capps, 1998, p. 80).

CHAMPIONING WOMEN'S ISSUES

According to a report by the National Women's Health Resource Center (1991), "Every six minutes, somewhere in this country, a woman is raped and every 15 seconds a woman will be beaten" (p. 6). In the United States in 1994 there were over 20,000 programs for battered women, the first shelter having opened just 20 years earlier (Diamond, 1994). The alarming and escalating rate of breast cancer is a social issue with significant impact on the lives of women. Also increasingly significant is the growing number of women experiencing coronary artery disease and myocardial infarction. The Roe v. Wade decision on abortion is being challenged regularly in the courts of many states across the nation. Eddie Bernice Johnson has sponsored or been involved in legislation on mammograms, maternity leave, and the right to choose abortion. Johnson has said:

All issues are women's issues. There are some issues that are women's business . . . there are some issues that I figure are my business. And choice is one of those. Mammograms and health care for women—these issues are my business. (Margolies-Mezvinsky, 1994, p. 95)

Consistent with Johnson's view and known health challenges confronting women daily, several of those interviewed identified very pressing issues of importance to women. Among these individuals were Eileen Cody, Marilyn Lee, Sharon Cooper, Joseph Polisena, and Maureen O'Connell. Women's issues they have chosen to focus on have included: breastfeeding in the workplace, economic and social issues, discriminatory practices by insurance companies in relation to family violence against women, stalking, "drive through" mastectomies and deliveries, partial-birth abortions (pro and con), and legislation for the court to impose consecutive sentences on serial rapists. O'Connell believes that "We've made great strides bringing political attention to the issue of breast cancer." She also plans to work on developing greater awareness about cardiovascular disease in women and this will be a "focus on the women's caucus for this year [1999], and on the health committee I will make that a priority also." Other issues being addressed are economic, including maternity leave, equal pay for equal work, and child care related to welfare reform to enable women to work when their welfare expires.

RESPONDING TO THE HIV/AIDS PANDEMIC

In 1994, the World Health Organization reported that the number of people worldwide who have AIDS was about 4 million (1994). The numbers have continued to grow, with 24 million cases reported in 1999 (Centers for Disease Control and Prevention, 1999). A Presidential Commission on the HIV epidemic, appointed by President Ronald Reagan in 1987, concluded that "if the generic problems in health care in the United States were not resolved, little could be done to contain the epidemic" (Ungvarski, 1995, p. 51). The nursing community was slow to respond up to that point, when the Association of Nurses in AIDS Care (ANAC) was formed as a way of "awakening the public as well as the nursing profession to the unique issues surrounding the epidemic" (Ungvarski, 1995, p. 51). This organization has come to represent the experts in the field.

   Prominent in leading the way in HIV/AIDS, Kristine Gebbie played a significant role in expanding public awareness of this pandemic. While serving as the National AIDS Policy Coordinator, she was responsible for educating federal employees, 3 million of them, about HIV/AIDS. She was instrumental in moving The White House to take a more proactive stance in AIDS awareness and education. This included President Clinton's breakfast meeting with the "faith community" and his establishment of the first AIDS Awareness Day. She brought to the table the need for research, for spending dollars wisely in balancing prevention and awareness, and the need for partnerships among agencies involved in these efforts. Gebbie responded to an incredible number of requests to speak out about HIV/AIDS, including schools, civic groups, and community organizations. Paula Hollinger, Patricia Vance, Judy Uherbelau, Maureen O'Connell, Mary Wakefield, and Barbara Wright have worked on AIDS legislation issues. These have included confidentiality, an AIDS notification law providing that no one is denied treatment because of this diagnosis and where those diagnosed are asked to identify their partners to facilitate early intervention, and an extension of the period of time in which New Jersey hemophiliacs who get AIDS can sue the pharmaceutical industry. In a consultant role, Wakefield worked with the World Health Organization to develop a global AIDS policy. Uherbelau "helped develop the county's first AIDS task force [in southern Oregon]" (Uherbelau, 1999, p. 14). According to Vance, Pennsylvania does not mandate recording of HIV, while 38 other states do. "I'm going to do that [bring the issue to the table]."

ADVANCING NURSING PRACTICE

Back in 1977, Marilyn Goldwater read an article in which two nurses said they were denied reimbursement from insurance companies for their practice. Her interest was piqued and she looked at what was taking place in her state of Maryland, where she found that nurse practitioners faced the same barrier. Following that, she crafted a bill to mandate reimbursement. She gathered "nurses and satisfied patients to testify in the bill's favor and otherwise support it, and circulated [sic] the bill to the insurance industry and physicians to learn how they'd argue against it" (Meyer, 1992, p. 58). Before the Maryland House Committee on

Economic Matters heard the bill, Goldwater worked out all the details with those individuals who would testify and discussed fully the arguments that could come up. At the hearing itself, she clearly showed the social force of nursing in a dramatic "bit of theater." She asked everyone present to stand if they supported the bill; all the nurses stood "wearing their uniforms and their stethoscopes and, believe me, it made quite a showing" (Meyer, 1992, p. 58). Following this, supporters fanned out in their communities to lobby their legislators. There were some rough hurdles along the way, and a compromise that included writing two different bills, one to cover nurse midwives and the other nurse practitioners. Goldwater reasoned that the former role, nurse midwives, was clearer for legislators to understand and would likely be easier to pass initially. She was right. The bill for reimbursement of nurse midwives passed both the house and senate and was signed by the governor of Maryland. With this precedent, Goldwater was able to move the nurse practitioner bill through the following year.

In 1997, the federal Balanced Budget Act gave nurse practitioners and clinical nurse specialists the right of direct reimbursement for services provided to Medicare beneficiaries in any setting. "Direct Medicare reimbursement for APNs [advanced practice nurses] is now a reality after years of lobbying" (Wong, 1999, p. 167). After a number of years of lobbying by organized nursing, advanced practice nurses are now defined by legislation as qualified providers. Wong cites two reasons that Congress acted favorably on this legislation: lack of access to cost-effective quality care, and the need for government to reduce the expenditures on Medicare (p. 169). This was well supported by the extant documentation about the quality of care by advanced practice nurses, including the finding by the congressional Office of Technology Assessment (OTA) that "NPs [nurse practitioners] can deliver as much as 80% of the health services, and up to 90% of pediatric care provided by primary care physicians, at equal to or better quality, and at lower cost (cited in American Association of Colleges of Nursing Media Backgrounder, April, 1998, p. 4). This landmark legislation has further legitimized the nurse as an independent health care practitioner and opened the door to additional initiatives in direct third-party reimbursement.

Nursing practice issues were on the agenda of the vast majority of those interviewed. Most had some involvement in policies
and legislation that involved the practice of nursing, from licensure laws concerned with scope of practice and titling issues, to
nurses' delegation, to continuing education on domestic violence.
In addition to Goldwater, perhaps some of the more involved in
this arena were Virginia Trotter Betts, Mary Wakefield, Sheila
Burke, Mary Moseley, Veronica Stephens, Nancy Valentine, Patricia
Montoya, and Eve Franklin. The issues they have brought to the
table have included: changing the traditional physician-based
model to a provider-based model, where "provider" includes
nurses and other appropriate health care practitioners; increasing
federal support for nursing education and research; third-party
reimbursement and prescriptive privileges; and addressing the
disparity between licensing and what nurses are prepared to do,
titling and scope of practice for advanced practice nurses, and
nurses' eligibility to open an Area Health Education Center
(AHEC). Wakefield said that she tries to articulate nursing's view
when she advocates dollars for nursing research and education.
She thinks that during the past 10 years more people have
begun to pay attention so that dollars are being allocated to
these areas.

SHAPING INSURANCE REFORM

Medicare, Medicaid, and HMO reforms were prominent topics
addressed by Sheila Burke, Allison Giles, Bonnie Ryan, Mel Callan,
Judy Uherbelau, Marilyn Goldwater, and other participants. From
the 1970s to the present, these women have had a hand in shaping legislation pertaining to medical/health insurance. Whether
drafting, sponsoring, or supporting legislation for reform, they
stayed their course. Their leadership was felt in terms of Medicare
and Medicaid, on issues such as hospice and home care coverage, small business implications of reform, and nursing home and
long-term care coverage. For example, Burke was involved from
1977 to 1996 in drafting Medicare, Medicaid, and national health
insurance legislation while on the staff of Senator Robert Dole
(R-Kansas). Giles commented on small business implications in
relation to President Bill Clinton's national health reform bill. She
participated in discussions about issues including confidentiality,

liability, and insurance coverage issues. Ryan brought together diverse people in the hospice community to restore hospice benefits for Medicaid patients in Illinois.

HMO reforms have been supported, in part, through the following initiatives: requirement to offer point-of-service plans and appeals procedures for HMO clients (according to Marilyn Goldwater, Maryland has one of the strongest procedures in the country). Uherbelau told of a bill that came up in 1997 involving full disclosure by HMOs on financial arrangements with physicians. The first time, the bill did not pass, but the second time it did, after everyone "worked together to pass the bill." Uherbelau worked on two HMO bills modeled after the one in Texas that provided for appeal to a third party and the ability to sue.

LEADING HEALTH CARE REFORM

Health care reform was the mantra of the 1990s. On the national agenda, supported by the American Nurses Association, state and district nurses associations, and individual nurses, health care reform as a national issue created a "face" for nursing at the national level. As a profession, nursing "joined the policy debate early with Nursing's Agenda for Health Care Reform (American Nurses Association [ANA], 1991) and continued as a visible player throughout the entire period" (Mundt, 1997, p. 19). The many debates about health reform resulted in multiple solutions, but relatively little in the way of outcomes at the national level.

The area of health reform was also on the agenda of many participants, including Eve Franklin, Claire Shulman, Lois Capps, Eddie Bernice Johnson, Mary McGrattan, and Barbara Wright. State and national health reform that increases access for all citizens is a commitment that was a prominent goal of those interviewed. Initiatives have included a model bill, the Managed Care Consumer Protection Act that is the first of its kind in the United States. This was developed during a "Women in Government" invitational meeting where there was representation from 10 states. As reported by Wright, this multi-state effort included a "no gag" rule. Another effort is the controversial national Patients' Bill of Rights of 1999 and the Patient Safety Act in Maryland. Advocating health insurance for the "working poor," individuals who are not eligible for Medicaid, is yet another effort toward health reform undertaken by McGrattan. On the topic of national health care, Johnson remarked, when interviewed, that paid advertisements in the mid-1990s distorted the picture of what national health care was about. The message served to create a great deal of doubt about the benefits of national health care. Also, people were afraid of change. "The status quo is easier for most people," said Johnson.

OTHER PRESSING SOCIAL ISSUES

There are numerous other far-reaching social issues that are being dealt with daily by appointed and elected officials and by those who campaigned and lost. These include education, unemployment, welfare reform, urban development, gun control, domestic violence, tax relief for big business, a "lemon law" for handicapped equipment (Rhode Island), taxes, designation of guide dogs as service animals that enables them to be in public places (Washington), victim's rights (Megan's Law, New Jersey), health education for schools, environmental safety, and placement of defibrillators in police cars (Rhode Island). In her role as Deputy Commissioner of Health, Donna Gentile O'Donnell has been involved in crime prevention measures. She teamed together police patrols and parole officers, knowing that parole officers have better access to criminals. She looked at the neighborhood of Philadelphia and the people who lived there. She found that citizens were most supportive of addressing the issue of crime, so she talked about crime prevention and looked at different models.

Education is another issue being addressed by a number of the people interviewed. For example, in discussing her work on the House of Representatives Education Committee Carolyn McCarthy said she had focused on "giving our teachers the best tools we can to teach our children." She has been involved in legislation that provides for a mentoring program where "more experienced teachers can help new recruits with any rough spots that come up during the day, and offer sound advice." The environment is an issue on the minds of many of the elected and appointed officials we interviewed. For example, Kay Khan described her interest in protecting the villages in her district. She meets with groups to talk about noise pollution and the effect of transportation on the environment. Through her work on the Community

Advisory Board, where she was chair for the last 4 of the 10 years she served, Marilyn Lee has been involved in zoning issues related to the building of roads and environmental safety. Muriel Shore said she was influential in moving the focus of government in New Jersey to the environment and quality of life issues.

SHOWING ONE'S FACE: IMPACT ON POLITICAL PROCESSES AND OUTCOMES

The accomplishments of these elected and appointed officials have been great. When asked to describe the impact they have made on political processes and outcomes, some were modest in attributing the impact to themselves; others readily claimed leadership in respect to the changes that occurred. One participant said that she sponsored several pieces of legislation, but that "none were earthshaking." Another was instrumental in getting legislation through, despite the fact that she was both a freshman legislator and a member of the minority party. Others depended on their relationships with state and national nursing associations to learn the issues, hear solutions, and rally support to move agendas forward. One participant responded to the question about impact by saying, "It depends if you ask on a good day or a bad day." Others spoke with pride about their accomplishments, some cautioning that, despite tangible progress, there are still many challenges ahead that require our attention. Although just a sampling, the following vignettes are a way to celebrate the impact of these nurses on social issues.

Beth Mazzella waxed eloquent on her work that began 30 years ago to establish the National Health Service Corps (NHSC) and the National Health Corps Scholarship Program. As a student, she was president of the National Student Nurses Association. She lobbied and testified on behalf of legislation to support the NHSC. As part of the National Urban Coalition, she lobbied to ensure that minorities, diversity, and "all those things we needed to care for those people were part of those programs, and 20 years later I was the administrator of that program." As Director of the NHSC Scholarship Program, she saw her dreams come to fruition. She said that it was interesting to sit there and be able to think about what it was she wanted to do as a student, not understanding how the process worked, but having a dream. "I think I am very fortunate to be able to say that I have made that kind of policy."

There's an issue that Mary McGrattan has had difficulty getting a "handle on," one that is not necessarily just a Connecticut issue. Simultaneous with being a legislator, she works in a long-term care facility, where she has observed that a lot of prescription drugs are "thrown out" when, for example, the drug becomes discontinued, or the resident has an allergic reaction. She has been told that "once a month the director or the assistant director of nursing at my work literally goes and gets a blender, blends up all the stuff, and flushes it down the toilet." They are allowed to return certain drugs, which becomes a "very laboring type of work." Another complicating factor is the bureaucracy. For example, if a drug is charged to one individual and half of it is returned, how does the charge get reconciled? She has been concerned with the waste of these drugs and consequent financial implications, and discussed the problem with the lieutenant governor of her state. Cost and licensure issues were then raised, but there was no receptivity to changing the way things are done. McGrattan brought this issue up once at a conference, and saw that this was a national issue not confined to Connecticut. While there continue to be many naysayers, she said that she intends to "keep hammering on" the path to change. Changing the status quo is never easy; however, through this process, she has raised awareness of the issue and caused others to question how they do business.

Eddie Bernice Johnson said she "paved the way for women to run for office." She began her career in public office in 1972 and is the first African American woman in Dallas to be elected to a public office. Her congressional biography states, "In the face of tremendous opposition, she ran as an underdog candidate, winning a landslide victory to the Texas House of Representatives. She was the first woman representing Dallas . . . since 1935." In addition to being the first nurse elected to serve in the United States House of Representatives in 1992, she is the first woman to have served from the state of Texas since Congresswoman Barbara Jordan in the 1970s. Although she has made great strides on behalf of women, she admits that there is still much work to be done to overcome the barriers—"old ways of thinking are still prevalent in many good people."

Joseph Polisena was a firefighter for 22 years. For 14 of those years he was at the same time a nurse. He was elected to his first 2-year term as a Rhode Island Senator in 1992, and was then re-elected in 1994. He chose not to run for a third term, but instead ran for mayor of his town. He lost the mayoral race, but plans to try to regain his state senate seat in the year 2000. Because he "learned how to deal with people [while a nursing student] and was knowledgeable on health care," he quickly became Deputy Majority Leader. During his brief time as a legislator, he sponsored or cosponsored more than 30 bills that became laws, and describes these as "mostly health bills." These have included mandatory stay for mastectomy (at least 48 hours), placement of defibrillators in police cars (the first state to do so), a lemon law for handicapped equipment, prescriptive privileges for nurse practitioners, and third-party reimbursement for nurse anesthetists. He was also a proponent of a health commission investigating a relationship between landfills and brain cancer that he said did not have definitive outcomes through this investigation.

Angela Uherbelau wrote an editorial that was published in *Newsweek* (see Appendix C) describing the negative campaigning faced by her mother, Judy Uherbelau, when she ran for the legislature in the state of Oregon. Uherbelau was portrayed by her opponent as anti-education, interested more about lawsuits than compassion, and worse! She wrote:

> Some may say that being Judy's daughter makes me unable to judge fairly any challenge to her ability as a legislator. I expect her opponent to take issue with her legislative record in order to point out clear differences between them. What I object to is having her record distorted to fit a sound bite or her entire life history twisted into a catch phrase. (Uherbelau, 1999, p. 14)

Fortunately, Angela wrote, smarter heads prevailed, as "supporters wrote letters to the newspapers condemning negative tactics and pointing out Mom's strengths as a legislator" (Uherbelau, p. 14). Due to term limits, Uherbelau will not be running in 2000; however, her daughter hopes that the candidates who campaign in the next election for her seat will "choose to run a clean and accurate campaign."

Christine Canavan said that in "every [legislative] session I have had success with something related to 'medical'," and states that being a nurse helped her to identify these problems. As a dialysis nurse, Canavan became aware of insurance and government regulations in terms of health care. In an outpatient facility where she worked, she saw that regulations were not being enforced and working conditions were unsafe, since nurses had to serve too many patients at the same time. She knew that reform was badly needed. One of the bills she sponsored in 1993 was the first bill filed in Massachusetts on patient care ratios. The bill mandates one direct care worker to three dialysis patients. She said that she didn't have to debate the merits of the bill because she is a nurse. In 1994 there was a resurgence of hepatitis B and tuberculosis. She was able to get a $100,000 grant to immunize teachers against hepatitis B in cases where insurance plans didn't cover immunization. She has been working with the Massachusetts Nurses Association on a whistleblower bill and on an HMO bill that is designed to reopen the conversation on managed care and return 90% of the profits to the customer and health care service.

Susan Reinhard has made a difference in the health and social policies of New Jersey, as prime mover of a number of bills with a clear voice of reason. Over the years she has advanced legislation on such issues as third-party reimbursement, school health, prescriptive privileges, and pronouncement of death, and has also advanced social consciousness in speaking on behalf of seniors. In recommending to the governor the merging of 20 programs from four departments to form the Department of Health and Senior Services, Reinhard put forth the desire to create a common value system and mission to promote "independence, dignity, and choice." As the highest-ranking nurse in the state, Reinhard has geared more senior services to being provided in the home; increased the allocation of dollars to fund home and community-based care by $60 million; gone to nursing homes to ascertain if people really want to be there (and helped them go home if they don't and are able to do so); and identified ways to decrease the burden of the family caregiver through respite care. She was a principal founder of the Governor's Nursing Merit Award to recognize the best and brightest nurses in New Jersey. A prolific writer and supporter of organized nursing, Reinhard shares her commitment to health and public policy with other nurses.

Bonnie Ryan's practice in oncology led her to directing a small hospice program in Chicago. She built the program "from the ground up," was recruited to develop a second, nursing home-based hospice, and then a third large integrated health care system hospice. She became involved with a state hospice organization and served on its board. She then was involved with a grassroots effort to lobby for restoration of the hospice Medicaid benefits in Illinois. Bringing together diverse people in the hospice community around a common cause, she was successful in restoring the hospice care benefit. She believed in what she was doing and "persevered despite great odds." When interviewed she asked, "What price will you pay to make a difference?" Subsequently, Ryan became involved in three state (Illinois, Indiana, and Wisconsin) public advocacy committees to work on hospice licensure, end-of-life legislation, and Medicaid reform. In her current position with the Veterans Administration (VA), she developed a national strategy for home and community-based hospice care based on the VA system. She also organized a national summit on end-of-life care. She was attracted to the VA because it was "undergoing massive change." She wanted to use her life experiences to make a difference in health care in her area of expertise.

Lieutenant Colonel Rosemary Nelson has spent 20 years in the Army. Based on her educational and experiential background in nursing informatics and management information systems, she has been involved in determining the qualitative and quantitative benefits of implementing technology in health care delivery. She was sent to Ft. Knox in 1988 to Composite Health Care Systems (CHCS), an alpha test site. Between 1991 and 1994 she served in a CHCS I Program Office and worked on a worldwide computerized patient record for the Department of Defense. This was a "showcase" for the Department, and Nelson went out on the lecture circuit. She was transferred to Europe with CHCS I where she was in Army facilities (hospitals and clinics) in Germany, Italy, and Belgium. This tour lasted 17 months, after which she returned to Washington DC's CHCS Program Office to become Deputy Program Manager. In late 1996, CHCS II was developed, and Nelson was involved in developing a longitudinal patient record that moves with the patient and managing a $250 million budget. She was again transferred, in 1998, to Honolulu as Program Manager and Chief Information Officer for the Pacific Rim (PERPO), where her work involves telehealth, telemedicine, clinical informatics research, and telehealth applications. In addition, she has been involved in demonstrating and validating commercial and emerging technology and in the assessment and testing of information technology to assure compliance for the year 2000. Her impact was in changing the general opinion of nurses by others. She feels that this kind of role needs nursing input and "know-how." A clinical focus is needed to deliver technology to the clinician, bringing the "user's voice to the table . . . We must groom clinical champions who can internalize and interpret technology . . . technology will be a way of life."

On a 2-year leave of absence from a tenured teaching position because her husband's job took them to Washington, DC, Mary Moseley decided to do something different. She felt that she wanted to address quality of life issues as a result of the changing American health care scene. Her entrée to the legislative offices of United States Senator Bill Frist (R-Tennessee), a physician, was through the front door—she just showed up—and she assumed a position as a fellow, then staff member. While there, the legislative director for the Public Health and Safety Committee initially assigned her to work on Title VIII of the United States Public Health Service Act. She started from scratch to get the bill together, working with a number of physicians. Her skills as a registered nurse were respected. Although nurses were never allowed to work on Title VII, since this was always within the purview of physicians and concerned Area Health Education Centers (AHECs), she went beyond working on Title VIII to Title VII, and in that way "helped get nurses in." Now nurses are eligible to open an AHEC. As a staff member, she also was instrumental in developing a Capitol Hill emergency plan. Here she worked alongside emergency physicians. During the time she was in this role, Moseley also worked one day a week as an instructor at a local college. She brought students to meet with Senator Frist to expose them to the political process and to mentor them. She feels strongly that you need to get students involved early if they are going to be involved.

A final vignette concerns Nancy Valentine. Always interested in leadership, she was even elected leader in grade school! While living in Pennsylvania, she received a master's degree in psychiatric nursing and business administration. She was a hospital administrator during the 1970s and never thought about politics. When she moved to Boston, she returned to school and attended the Harvard School of Public Health. There were only two or three nurses in the program, who found themselves in the position of "breaking down the gender barrier." Following this, she received a fellowship through the Department of Health and Human Services, where she was mentored in government roles. For a long time, Valentine has "helped set policies in male-dominated organizations," where nursing was controlled by medicine. She created a policy shift. In 5 years, 35 Veterans Administration nurses moved from a subservient role to a Vice President role. Nurses felt that "the barrier had been lifted." Nursing was seen in a different light within the organization. She next looked at research funding, and discovered that VA nurses had the ability to do research but did not have the resources to do so. Through the new Undersecretary of Health, a nursing research project was created with substantial funding for nursing research. Valentine considers this a major breakthrough. In addition, she was successful in expanding the work and workforce of advanced practice nurses at the VA, the first national distance learning program offered through the Uniform Services University, including credentialing requirements for upward mobility of nurses within the VA system. On the latter outcome, she "mounted a long and tedious process looking at experiences in the private and public sectors regarding outcomes based on credentials." She had to deal with unions that opposed requiring higher degree credentials and partnered with universities around the country to raise the level of education of VA nurses. Over time she was able to gain union support and secure $50 million to assist VA nurses to move along the educational continuum. While she recognizes that not all VA nurses will move into baccalaureate and master's programs, she "would like to see the path made easier for them." Valentine was effective in her role by bringing information to the table and being "articulate about what the trends and shortfalls were."

It is indeed exciting to bask in the light of these significant changes that have occurred in our social fabric as a result of the actions of these and many other nurses. We should not forget, though, that we are merely on the cusp of what can be. The future impact of nurses in addressing social issues depends largely on keeping our "faces" out front, where both colleagues and the public can see and can benefit from our commitment. Chapter 5, Negotiating the Political Process, and chapter 6, Creating Political Opportunities, provide some insights to start on this path.

REFERENCES

American Association of Colleges of Nursing Media Backgrounder: Nurse Practitioners. (1998, April). Washington, DC: American Association of Colleges of Nursing.

American Nurses Association. (1991). *Nursing's agenda for health care reform.* Kansas City, MO: Author.

An interview with Mary K. Wakefield, PhD, RN, FAAN (1992, May). *Healthcare Trends & Transition, 3*(6), 14–17.

Atwood, K., Colditz, G. A., & Kawachi, I. (1997). From public health science to prevention policy: Placing science in its social and political contexts. *American Journal of Public Health, 87*(10), 1603–1606.

Capps, L. (1998). Nurses' voices needed in halls of Congress. *American Journal of Nursing, 98*(9), 80.

Centers for Disease Control and Prevention (1999). *HIV/AIDS Surveillance Report, 10*(2), 1–43.

Deets, C. (1999). Research: Too little too late? *Journal of Professional Nursing, 15*(4), 80.

Diamond, K. (1994, April 21). Society's role in stopping domestic violence. *Staten Island Advance,* C2.

Dreamer, O. M. (date unknown). *The invitation.*

FY2000 President's Budget Press Briefing. Available online: http://www4.od.nih.gov/ofm/budget/fy2000pressbriefing.htm.

Glass, L. K. (1984, December). Safeguarding society's welfare: Nursing's political history. *Nursing Success Today, 1*(4), 39–40.

Gretter, L. (1993). Address of President Lystra Gretter. In N. Birnbach & S. Lewenson (Eds.), *Legacy of leadership: Presidential addresses from the Superintendents' Society and the National League of Nursing Education 1894–1952* (pp. 44–52). New York: National League for Nursing Press. (Original work published 1902)

Henderson, V. (1960). *Textbook of the principles and practice of nursing.* New York: Macmillan.

Kitson, A. L. (1997). Johns Hopkins address: Does nursing have a future? *Image: Journal of Nursing Scholarship, 29*(2), 111–115.

Labelle, H. (1986). Nurses as a social force. *Journal of Advanced Nursing, 11,* 247–253.

Malone, B. L., & Keepnews, D. (1998). Ensuring the future of nurses in clinical practice: Issues and strategies for staff nurses and advanced practice nurses. In D. Mason & J. K. Leavitt (Eds.), *Policy and politics in nursing and health care* (3rd ed., pp. 294–306). Philadelphia: W. B. Saunders.

Margolies-Mezvinsky, M. (1994). *A woman's place . . . The freshmen women who changed the face of Congress.* New York: Crown.

Mason, D., Cohen, S. S., O'Donnell, J., Baxter, K., & Chase, A. (1997). Managed care organizations' arrangements with nurse practitioners. *Nursing Economic$, 15*(6), 306–314.

Meyer, C. (1992, October). Nursing on the political front. *American Journal of Nursing, 92,* 56–64.

Mundt, M. H. (1997). Books on health policy and health reform: How is nursing represented? *Journal of Professional Nursing, 13*(1), 19–27.

National Women's Health Resource Center. (1991). *Violence against women: Report of the June 21, 1991 conference.* Washington, DC: Author.

Saslow, L. (1999, August 15). Going into sticker shock at the drugstore. *The New York Times,* Section 14, pp. 1, 15.

Uherbelau, A. (1999, March 29). My turn: Is this a job worth fighting (fair) for? *Newsweek,* p. 14.

Ungvarski, P. J. (1995). HIV/AIDS: Lessons learned from an epidemic. *Journal of the New York State Nurses Association, 26*(1), 51–53.

Wallace, D. C., McGuire, S. L., Lee, H. T., & Sauter, M. (1999). Older Americans Act: Implications for nursing. *Nursing Outlook, 47*(4), 181–185.

Wong, S. T. (1999). Reimbursement to advanced practice nurses (APNs) through Medicare. *Image: Journal of Nursing Scholarship, 31*(2), 167–173.

World Health Organization. (1994, July 1). *The current global situation of the HIV/AIDS pandemic* (Press Release). Geneva, Switzerland: Author.

Negotiating the Political Process: Lessons Learned

> Courage, that we may bravely face the difficulties yet to be overcome, recognizing that these are meant to arouse not to discourage, "that even defeat is nothing but education, nothing but the first to something better," and "failures with heroic minds are the stepping stones to success."
>
> —Snively

Serving the public has been described as a privilege and an honor. People seek public office and political appointments for many reasons. Power, status, and money are among the reasons often associated with politicians who serve; however, the nurses interviewed gave different reasons. They saw themselves as making a change, creating a better environment, doing nursing on a larger scale, or being part of the community, but not as politicians. They brought their ideals from their past, whether there was something they learned in nursing or from their personal life, and translated it into their role as an elected official or a political appointee. The people who decided to run felt a compelling need to offer their service. Some of those interviewed "fell" into their positions, while others chose their political course deliberately. They all described how they willingly gave their time, expertise, and energy. Most described the extraordinary amount of time they gave to public service. It was a major commitment and one that required stamina of all involved, and one that was at times all-consuming. Eddie Bernice Johnson said, "Nurses are workaholics. They need to be scheduled to stop!" This may be among the more important lessons to be learned.

This chapter describes some of the lessons learned by these 40-plus nurses who ran for public office and won, who served as appointed officials, or who ran and lost. The lessons varied from person to person, but many shared common experiences. Many of the lessons learned, such as giving enormous personal investment of time, being part of a grassroots efforts, claiming their nursing identity, broadening their horizons, asking for money, learning who they are, and surviving the sometimes cutthroat nature of politics, have shaped the experiences of those individuals. No doubt, these lessons will continue to shape the strategies that nurses will use in the future.

LESSON 1: IT TAKES A PERSONAL INVESTMENT

Candidates found that running for public office required a tremendous personal investment in terms of time. Prior to the election, all of a candidate's time is devoted to campaign activities. Pat Latona said she stood outside freezing in the predawn hour of 6:00 A.M. to hand out fliers and shake hands. You've got to meet the voters where they work, live, and commute! Standing by train stations or supermarkets and shaking hands are all part of the time-consuming campaign activities. You also need to be prepared with an extraordinary amount of information about local issues as well as broader, more global ones. People will ask you questions, and you need to know how broader issues will affect them in your own home state and town. Many told us that during a campaign, you must be ready to give your time and personal space to get your name out there. They told us that they walked door to door campaigning. Interestingly enough, many of the nurses who had public health backgrounds felt they were good at door-to-door, because that is what they had always done in nursing. Stopping in to ask how someone was doing, caring, and being there for them, even for a short time, won votes.

Interfacing with the public after being elected, as well as before, means that you attend meetings, sometimes two and three on a Saturday and Sunday; you attend public hearings, go to soccer games, attend walkathons, and appear at fundraising events. One of the participants noted that she no longer had much private time. Even with reserving Sunday for her family, she found herself approached by her constituents and supporters while at church. Every night she attended at least two affairs and four on the weekends. She explained, "Your time is not your own."

The notion that your time is not your own repeated itself in most of the interviews. Montana State Legislator Eve Franklin described that she was "truly a public servant." Having no office or staff, she was frequently called at home. She saw herself as being "owned" by her constituents. While the expectations of her role sometimes left her feeling particularly challenged, she emphatically noted that nothing ever stopped her. She worked long and hard to make the changes she thought were necessary.

LESSON 2: IT TAKES A GRASSROOTS EFFORT

Nurses in political office or who were politically appointed to a position often achieved their status by starting at the grassroots level. They began their campaign knocking on doors, volunteering in the community, serving on local town boards, or rallying around a particular issue. Nurses are trusted in the community, and support is readily given if they make themselves known. Judy Uherbelau worked on community projects as a child and continued in that vein as she grew up. Joining the Newton Democratic City Committee enabled Kay Khan to help local candidates win office. Her efforts on these campaigns subsequently gave her the visibility she needed to lead her own successful political career. Her deep interest in gaining third-party reimbursement for nurses and her pro-choice stand led her to seek public office.

"Its tough to beat a nurse," reasoned Judy Robson (1998, p. 426) during her campaign for a seat in the Wisconsin Assembly. Robson needed to overcome a strong, visible opponent and had to make herself known. Harnessing the energy of the Wisconsin State Nurses' Association, her professional colleagues, and student nurses, they called themselves the "white-shoe army" and campaigned for Robson. Patricia Vance became involved in her community by volunteering as a committeewoman on town boards. She noted that nursing skills were easily transferable to those needed in politics. "It's just a people thing, and politics really is a people business." If you are *not* good with people, you probably should not be in either nursing or politics.

Grassroots campaigning requires targeting the right groups to work on specific legislation. Mary Moseley, former aide to Senator Bill Frist, one of the few physicians in the Senate, advised us that is never too late to be schooled in grassroots lobbying efforts. What you need first is to know how bills become laws. Nurses should write letters, use data to support what they say, knock on doors, and be in constant contact with their legislators. Nursing educators need to get students involved early and include grassroots lobbying efforts in their curriculum. Moseley also learned that nurses need to spend more time mentoring each other.

LESSON 3: IT TAKES A NURSE

Their nursing backgrounds influenced the candidates, elected officials, and appointees. Being a nurse gave them credibility with the public. Although the public trusts nurses, we know that relatively few nurses hold office. Many of the nurses interviewed learned during the process of getting elected or appointed that they needed to capitalize on the trusted position nurses held in the public eye. They found that on the whole nurses were perceived by the public as honest, caring, and well respected, unless, as Pat Latona noted, their constituents had received bad nursing care.

When Cindy Empson from Kansas spoke with her constituents, she noted that they expected honesty from her because she was a nurse. Getting elected or appointed was the ultimate goal for many of these leaders, and it was important to recognize the value that being a nurse could bring to the success of their campaign. Iowa legislator Beverly Nelson-Forbes explained that she plays the political game by "telling it like it is." She said she was not much of a politician to start with, but she was "dead honest and a hard worker." She went on to say, "People know if they give me something to do they know it will get done." This kind of follow-through is certainly an essential nursing skill.

Nurses need to capitalize on this public trust to gain entry into the political arena. Some candidates, such as Christine Canavan, Paula Hollinger, and Margaret Leonard, included their RN credential on their campaign materials. Most of those who ran for office said that they told people they were nurses, and usually campaigned with their nursing identity close at hand. Connecticut State Legislator Mary McGrattan said that being from a small town, everyone knew she was a nurse. While she didn't always advertise the fact, her constituents knew. In her last election, McGrattan said, "the fact that I am an RN gave me some credibility to my position on managed care." She explained that when people associated her with being a nurse, they felt that she knew what she was talking about. Her expertise was trusted.

Congresswoman Lois Capps includes the statement that she is a nurse in her speeches. She is proud to be a nurse and uses her background wherever she can. The day before being interviewed for the book, Capps explained she had been sworn in as a member of the Unites States House of Representatives. She said she was overwhelmed by the tremendous support she had received as a nurse and felt a strong sense of camaraderie with the nurses who attended the swearing-in. Mary Wakefield described how when she worked for Senator Kent Conrad (D-North Dakota), he introduced her as his "chief of staff, who was a nurse and had a PhD." Wakefield explained that she liked this introduction, not because of the visibility for her, since she already had the job, but because it was important visibility for nurses. "Yes, this is something nurses can do and do effectively and something a United States Senator takes pride in." Wakefield believes that nurses are part of the solution, but the question is do we make that pitch. People often asked Wakefield why she left nursing. She viewed it differently, that she didn't leave nursing. In fact, she has used nursing and the skills learned in the profession and applied them to crisis management, problem solving, and informing health care policies.

While many of the nurses interviewed felt their constituents trusted nurses, these same constituents often did not know what nurses could offer in the political arena. It has been up to nurses to educate the public about the scope of nursing practice, the educational background of nurses, and the practice, educational, and research issues in which the profession is involved. Nurses have a great deal to offer in the way of expertise in health-related matters, and are clearly needed in the local, state, and national legislative bodies, as well as in appointed public positions.

One of the unexpected lessons learned by Kay Khan was that the nursing community had not taken advantage of her position in the Massachusetts State Legislature. It seemed surprising to her that more nurses in the state did not avail themselves of her services as legislator. While many nurses in our sample received a great deal of support from their state nurses associations, a few did not. One person said that she did not want the support of the nurses of her state, because of their lack of sophistication in lobbying and their boorish reactions when dealing with legislators that did not agree with them. Booing at legislators and writing nasty letters does not help you successfully achieve your goals. This nurse remarked that a spoonful of sugar will get you more. Nurses need to learn how to politically advocate change in ways that can be heard. In order to be included at the policymaking table, we need to be able to negotiate, listen, and debate the points we want to make.

One of the most interesting responses to the question of whether people saw them differently because they were nurses came from Beverly Nelson-Forbes. She raised the issue of the difficulty of being a woman in the legislature, a historically male bastion of power. Nelson-Forbes said,

> I think it is more that you're a woman and have to find your place
> . . . I think they respect you for the fact that you're a professional
> and that you're a nurse probably more so than their respect for
> women legislators.

The male legislators who were in the majority respected the professional side of the nurse; however, they had more difficulty with the idea of a woman serving in office. Women legislators have to find their place as women.

It takes a nurse to cut through rigid positions on some of the most compelling social issues. One such issue concerns abortion. While most of those interviewed supported pro-choice for women, a small minority did not. In speaking about women in Congress, Eddie Bernice Johnson (Margolis-Mezvinsky, 1994) was quoted as having said, "We can't assume that every woman will come in the same frame of mind. I have watched facial expressions when choice comes up and I can't even imagine a woman—and I've never had a desire for an abortion and I grew up basically in the Catholic Church—but I cannot even imagine a woman not wanting to have some say over her body" (pp. 95–96). One individual who supported pro-life, however, did so with the caveat that being a nurse tempered her position on the subject. Sharon Cooper said that being a nurse provided her with a different perspective from her colleagues in the legislature. While she is a pro-life advocate, she is a realist and doesn't expect that the law will change; however, she would like to see the least number of abortions performed. Her nursing background and life experiences support this position. She had attended a Catholic nursing school at a time when abortion was illegal. While this background may have shaped her opposition to pro-choice, she had seen two deaths from illegal abortions and this, she believes, tempers things for her.

LESSON 4: IT TAKES A BROADER VIEW THAN NURSING

In agreement with many of the other nurses interviewed, Mary Wakefield said that we must broaden our horizons and not just talk "nurse speak." While we need to identify ourselves as nurses, we need to demonstrate a wider breadth of knowledge. Wakefield explained that her ability to talk about other fields gave her an entrée. Whether she was talking with the Governor of the State or someone from General Electric, if she had things to say other than nursing, concerning either health care more broadly or other current events, she could engage the individuals on their own turf. By doing so, people recognized that she was paying attention to issues that went beyond nursing and health care. They were then more willing to pay attention to her concerns about nursing and health care policy.

"You cannot rely just on your nursing background to see you through. You've got to know all the issues that face a community. When you do not know an issue, you sometimes get caught stumbling," said Pat Latona. You must do your homework and need to know more than just the local issues. Beverly Nelson-Forbes had to learn about issues that she had never thought existed. For example, one of the most emotional issues in her state this past year had to do with dove hunting. She received over 500 letters, telephone calls, and e-mails on the subject. Hunters wanted to go out and "shoot those poor little doves." Doves, she learned, had a very short lifespan, living only a few months, and she noted,

"Everybody likes to wake up and hear the doves on a summer morning." While she felt that other issues such as education, highways, and lowering taxes might have been more pressing, all she heard about were the doves. She had to respond to her constituency and had to learn about the issues surrounding dove hunting. She hoped, however, that they did not have to take a vote on the subject because she knew she would make some of her constituents very unhappy.

Sometimes referred to as "the 101st Senator" (DeParle, 1995) while chief of staff to Senator Bob Dole (R-Kansas), Sheila Burke was involved in a wide range of issues requiring a broad view as well as a great deal of negotiating and "deal-making." One such issue was the welfare reform bill that was the focal point of federal legislation in the mid-1990s.

> With or without a family cap, the welfare bill that cleared the Senate with 87 votes topped off a stunning rush to the right. In ending poor children's entitlement to Federal aid, it struck a deathblow to 60 years of established social policy. And for better or worse, Burke helped wield the ax. (DeParle, 1995, p. 35)

Another issue Burke dealt with is the line item veto bill. She played an important role in getting this legislation through the Senate.

LESSON 5: IT TAKES POWER

The issue of being a woman, and the question that it raises in terms of power, had a strong influence on some of the nurses we interviewed that held office or an appointed position. Being a woman, as one of the legislators mentioned earlier in this chapter, was a harder barrier to overcome than being a nurse. In her book *A Woman's Place . . . The Freshmen Women Who Changed the Face of Congress,* Congresswoman Marjorie Margolies-Mezvinsky (1994) wrote,

> When we [freshmen women] arrived in Washington, we . . . expected to be challenged on a host of levels. We did not expect to be patronized or to be the victims of irritating and demeaning expressions of sexism . . . Instead of being confronted with legislative challenges, the first thing we had to worry about was being *recognized* as members of Congress. (p. 40)

Most nurses are women, and all but one of the nurses we interviewed were women. Many told us that frequently they were the only nurses on policymaking committees and were sometimes the only woman as well. The ways that women respond to and wield power become important for us to examine.

Nurses often claim a sense of powerlessness in their personal and professional lives. Ashley (1973) noted that this sense of powerlessness is predicated on the belief that someone else is in power. When Ashley wrote in the early 1970s, a time in which the women's movement made tremendous strides, she found few, if any articles in the literature that highlighted the "positive aspects of nursing power" (p. 637). Over a decade later, Hanley (1987) noted that the literature reflected an increase in women's participation in political activities. Hanley observed that women with higher education and who were employed were more likely to engage in political activities. She further noted that the amount of participation was related to the profession that employed them. For example, women working in male-dominated professions were more likely to adopt the political behaviors of the men in that field because this behavior was expected and rewarded. On the other hand, women situated in female-dominated professions were less politically active because of the lack of "defined resources of power, status, and prestige" (Hanley, 1987, p. 180). More than two decades after Ashley's writing, Winter and Lockhart (1997) more encouragingly noted that political activity could overcome the powerlessness expressed by some nurses. They saw an increase in this activity, an opinion which was supported in the nurses we interviewed. While they, too, struggled with the concept of power, the very activity of running for office, or serving in high governmental positions, allowed them to "do something" and to be in a position to make a change.

If, as McClure (1985) noted, power is something that nurses in the past have been "loathe to discuss" (p. 55) and it is regarded as a pejorative, then perhaps this explains nurses' reticence to run for office or, even when in office, why they shy away from claiming the limelight. One person we interviewed said that even though a lot of politicians in her area liked to get their name in the paper, she more felt comfortable spending her time accomplishing the things she did, and didn't need to "blow her own horn." Some of the nurses supported this notion, saying that they, too, liked to work in the background and leave the "politicking" for others. They felt that as nurses they liked to accomplish and complete tasks. When they introduced a bill they liked to see it through, and they encouraged people to call on them to solve problems and answer questions. Another nurse said she felt that she didn't lie to her constituents as some politicians did because she felt it was disgusting and her ego didn't need it.

Power relies on knowing what needs to happen and how to go about making it happen. Wielding power to make legislative change requires a strong sense of self that women, and more specifically nurses, do not always possess. Maraldo (1985) said that "Nurses lack the basic fundamental source of power, self-confidence" (p. 71). The fact that the nurses who were interviewed were actively engaged in the political process, however, indicates a feeling of empowerment and a shift away from some of the powerlessness that nurses feel. Yet more work needs to be done within our schools and practice settings to foster self-confidence and empower people.

A number of nurses interviewed believed that knowledge translated into power. Nancy Valentine, Special Assistant to the Undersecretary for Health, became more politically aware and active as she advanced her education with a master's degree in psychiatric nursing from University of Pennsylvania, and a master's degree in business administration from the Wharton School of Business. She later attended the Harvard School of Public Health. Following her experience at Harvard, Valentine received a fellowship through the Department of Health and Human Services, where she was mentored in a role in government. Her interest in policymaking continued as she worked as the Director of Nursing at Boston City Hospital. As a result of her work as an administrator of a hospital, Valentine became involved in city politics. She merged her interest in politics with her doctoral work, which she completed at Brandeis University in health policy and economics. While she had not started out thinking of politics, Valentine acknowledged that she moved her career in that direction gaining the knowledge and skills that put her in a position to be noticed, and subsequently sought after, for powerful appointed positions.

Power comes from knowing what needs to be changed as well as knowing the process to make change. Bonnie Ryan, Chief of the Veterans Administration Home and Community-Based Care, has the confidence to believe her work is important and is willing to persevere despite great odds. Success, Ryan said, is reinforcing. The more success in changing policy or influencing political agendas, the more likely it is that you will continue to do so. Ryan, however, looks at the downside of power that can accompany the successful accomplishment of change:

> The successes are really wonderful when you do make a difference. It's pretty exciting, and that in itself is dangerous, because power is very intoxicating and heady, and you can lose your balance very easily when you're in a strong position as well as when you're in a weak position.

Eve Franklin draws strength from realistically assessing how change is made and how to use the inherent power she has by virtue of her profession and her role as a Montana State Legislator. She said that the legislative process "is 50% theatre, 40% interpersonal skills, and 10% fact." This understanding helps her to direct some of her actions and to make change. A number of the nurses interviewed recognized the need to work within this kind of setting and formed coalitions with other groups such as women's caucuses. These groups helped them be successful in the "theater" and enabled them to use their interpersonal skills and knowledge in a constructive way to affect change.

LESSON 6: IT TAKES A THICK SKIN

Politics is often described as being "cutthroat" and a dangerous place to be. In our graduate classes on health care policy, students have described politicians using words such as "cigar-smoking," "slippery," "shady," and "stab-you-in-the-back kind of characters." Students have envisioned that deals are made in smoke-filled, back rooms where money is the bottom line. Working with politicians has been considered akin to swimming in shark-infested waters; one needs to be careful.

Indeed, there is much precedent for this perception (Margolies-Mezvinsky, 1994), and, in fact, the notion of the danger associated with politics was acknowledged by some of the nurses interviewed. For example, Imogene King reported having to deal with "dirty politics" played out in her small community. She had to overcome the effects of bad press, including a white paper with gross inaccuracies about her, by rallying her supporters and publishing her own white paper in response. Nancy Valentine recognized the need to have "thick skin," especially when you are not popular with the people with whom you would like to be popular. Valentine noted that she had "tenacity and perseverance" to see the job through. She felt these are two qualities that are needed in public service. Likewise, Eileen Cody noted that you need a "thick skin" for politics, a characteristic she believes is needed in nursing as well.

Kay Khan described politics as a very personal matter: What you are able to accomplish has to do with the relationships you establish, and especially with how you develop them and how you keep them. To connect with other legislators, Khan joined the women's caucus and established close ties with that group. She has learned that a "relational atmosphere" exists in Congress, and most politicians are relational kinds of people. Khan further reflected that a lot of what you do in politics has to do with "perseverance, and a willingness to just keep fighting, keep going, keep pushing, and recognizing that you're there to represent your community. They sent you up there to do certain things and you just do it. And to not take things personally and just do what you need to do."

The job of running for office or serving as an elected or appointed official requires a personal and professional commitment to being exposed and critiqued at all times. Whether in the supermarket, church, or gym, you may be called upon to respond to a constituent's request or may find yourself as the brunt of an unpleasant headline. Sheila Burke found herself embroiled in a smear campaign against her by right-wing conservatives. On November 12, 1995, *The New York Times* ran a story, "Sheila Burke is the Militant Feminist Commie Peacenik Who's Telling Bob Dole What to Think," in which the author, Jason DeParle, presents Burke as the "latest victim of the conservative attack machine" (p. 32). DeParle wrote that the "bashing of Burke is one of those modest, passing events that suddenly reveal a complex mix of the city's political morés" (p. 34). In the article, Burke was accused of being a "militant feminist," "former liberal Democrat" and "Hillary-Lite." DeParle quoted her response to some of these slurs as "I'm strong willed and I'm independent, and I see women as fully capable as men of doing anything they choose. I'm not in the least apologetic about any of that" (p. 34). Burke found herself misquoted and misrepresented, but also gained the support of several senators. For example, Senator John McCain (R-Arizona) was quoted as saying, "I don't know whether Sheila Burke is liberal, conservative, libertarian, or vegetarian—I know she is honest, decent, and hard working" (DeParle, 1995, p. 36).

Other nurses shared with us the need to be willing to open yourself up for comment and critique. Your life is on view, and you need to learn how to roll with the punches. Shirley Chater described the process in which she was confirmed as the Commissioner of the United States Social Security Administration as very intense, "so much so, that it can dissuade people from serving or entering public service." For her appointment, she had to undergo FBI checks, complete numerous, time-consuming financial forms, and have her family situation investigated, including her values and character.

LESSON 7: IT IS DIFFICULT TO LOSE

Those who lost ran campaigns similar to their nursing colleagues who won. They gave no less time, money, energy, and expertise than those who were successful in their election bids. They lost because they faced a strong opponent, had insufficient funds, had little or no name recognition, or were running on the wrong party line for that election. Although the reasons varied, none of the candidates interviewed felt that their unsuccessful campaigns were unsuccessful from lack of trying. They all shared the lessons they learned from their more successful counterparts. They just had to learn one more lesson: how to lose.

It is difficult to lose. Pat Latona, a Democrat from New York State, said she was devastated when she lost in a highly contested election. Three people had run for the same position on the Town Board in Mamaroneck, New York. The board was packed with Democrats, and voters that year were looking for a change. Her friend, a Republican and her opponent, won by 50 votes. Throughout the campaign, Latona raised money and organized many of the political events. During her campaign she did everything from attending debates and forums, to walking miles and miles, to knocking on doors, to going to every fair and soccer game she could attend. She spent most of her evenings after work and her weekends campaigning while her husband stayed at home with their children. It was a family affair, and one in which Latona worked long hours to win. The campaign consumed tremendous time and energy, but she felt she could make a difference. Latona explained that you must be committed to run. You develop an incredible wealth of knowledge that keeps building the more you are "out there" responding to the public. When asked if she would ever run again, she said, "Never say never."

LESSON 8: IT TAKES A POLITICAL PARTY

To get on the ballot and to get support usually requires a party affiliation. The candidates who ran for office recognized the importance of this backing. Barbara Wright changed her political affiliation to enter the Assembly race in New Jersey. Until 1986, after holding a 2-year position as Mayor of Plainsboro, New Jersey, Wright was a Democrat. She then decided not to affiliate with any party. This lasted 6 years until James Florio ran for Governor. She did not support Florio's platform, but was impressed by and wanted to work with Christine Todd Whitman. She decided to get back into the political arena and her friends told her, "If you can't get on the Democratic ticket then ask the Republicans to nominate you." So she changed her affiliation to the Republican Party. Likewise, Carolyn McCarthy made a switch. She said,

> Actually I am a registered Republican. I tried to run as a Republican, but the Republican Party on Long Island wouldn't let me run. So, never one to be deterred once I've made up my mind, I called the Democratic Party and they were happy to have me. So I ran on the Democratic ticket and won.

Those interviewed who held appointed positions generally said that they avoided any kind of partisan politics. They needed to remain neutral and apolitical; however, they felt they could still get their ideas across. Shirley Chater was an Independent, which she thought was an advantage when being considered in 1993 for the appointment to the Social Security Administration. The American Nurses Association lobbied hard during the Clinton administration to get appointments for nurses, and Dr. Chater was heavily backed by this organization. Some appointment "marriages" were from opposite parties. For example, Mary Moseley, a registered Democrat, worked for Senator Bill Frist (R-Tennessee). She said that health care is nonpartisan. Sheila Burke was a registered Democrat when she started working for Senator Bob Dole (R-Kansas). Interestingly enough, some of those who held a particular party affiliation retained their appointments even when the "reigning" party in office changed. The assumption here is that their values surpassed party lines.

LESSON 9: IT TAKES A MENTOR (OR DOES IT?)

Mentors often provide support and guidance in uncharted waters. Most of the nurses could point to mentors along the way. Some were the faculty they had in school; for others, it was a family member or close friend. Although in previous chapters mentoring relationships were mentioned, because this lesson is so critical, mentoring bears further emphasis here. Virginia Trotter Betts recalls that she had several mentors, including her nursing colleagues, faculty, fellow students, family, and her friends. Lois Capps found that other women in the Congress served as excellent mentors. She also noted that she has had men as well as women as mentors and has felt supported along the way. Eileen Cody can point to another nurse legislator in her state that served as mentor. Nurses who are elected, Cody remarked, should mentor other nurses and women in this role. Others, like Shirley Chater, had had mentors since their days in undergraduate nursing school. For example, Chater's Dean at the University of Pennsylvania, Theresa Lynch, served as her mentor during her undergraduate education, and Helen Nahm, Dean at UCSF was her mentor when she studied for her master's degree. In identifying her mentor, Kristine Gebbie pointed to the assistant director of her nursing program, Helen Hansen, who was also on the board of the *American Journal of Nursing* Company. Gebbie said, "To be any kind of nurse you need to be involved in your professional organization." Through these ties come relationships with strong mentors. Patricia Montoya said that she learned through observation, mentoring, general learning, and early and quick successes.

Many of the people interviewed agreed that mentoring was important to their growth, but they had to take a moment to reflect on who had mentored them along the way. A few said they had never thought about this before, noting that they learned as they went along. Some shared that they had just "stumbled" into everything, including their mentors. Allison Giles said that her mentor had taught her to be more aggressive and assertive than she thought she was by nature. Eddie Bernice Johnson felt that a number of people, rather than one particular individual, were available to "run things by," to come up with ideas, and to give her feedback. While not having a mentor to help make the decision to run for office, Judy Uherbelau spoke of her predecessor as her mentor. Until her mentor died, she gave Uherbelau tremendous support. Others, such as Marilyn Goldwater, felt that not enough mentoring went on. Once elected, she said, you learn your way around, making friends and learning from them. She could not recall a nurse that served as a mentor, and while several women legislators provided the guidance, they did so only in the beginning. Joseph Polisena said he did not have a mentor; rather, he did it on his own. Claire Shulman, as well, could not identify a specific mentor who was influential.

The mentors identified provided a myriad of support. Pat Latona's mentors were her teachers in graduate school. They helped shape her leadership skills by "pushing the envelope" and highlighting her positive qualities. Margaret Leonard's daughter, a political science major in college, mentored her during her campaign. Susan Reinhard said she never did anything alone. She always had mentors, including Assemblywoman Barbara Wright. Wright was also a mentor to Muriel Shore. Reinhard said that even with the mentors she had, she frequently learned from her mistakes. For example, she learned the hard way that inviting Democrats to a Republican fundraiser didn't work. Bonnie Ryan's mentor, Betty Cody, "opened new doors" for her. She took her by the hand and led her into an arena that she might not have entered otherwise by creating a "nurturing environment." Mary Simmons spoke of her mother's mentorship, encouraging in her a lifelong commitment to volunteerism. Her mother told her she "could be

anything and do anything she wanted" and this advice has
served her well. Cindy Empson looked at people she respected
and tried to pattern herself on their ideas.

Mary Wakefield described a few people who helped to launch
her career. One of them was the Executive Director of the North
Dakota State Nurses Association. When Wakefield applied for her
position in government, her mentor was extremely helpful, because
she personally knew the senator who would be interviewing her.
She was influential and a good person to learn from as she came
up from the ranks through the State Nurses Association. Another
person to mentor her growth was Billye Brown, former Dean of
the University of Texas in Austin, who gave advice, spent time,
and was positive and supportive. But when it came to mentors in
nursing on Capitol Hill early on, there weren't any for Wakefield.
She explained,

> So it was really more with the people I was working with on the Hill
> who took me under their wings, and they said this is how it works.
> So [it was] non-nurses basically, because there weren't any nurses
> in those jobs, or very few, and I didn't know where they were when
> I first got there.

Mentors can serve as role models and leaders. The majority of
those interviewed, regardless of whether or not they had a mentor, expressed the need for role models and mentors in policymaking and political positions. Since there are relatively few nurses
who seek and hold these kinds of positions, there are few mentors to support nurses interested in pursuing these avenues.
Bonnie Ryan said that as nurses we should do more mentoring.
We need to nurture our future political leaders. Many participants noted that schools of nursing need to include policymaking and political activism in their curricula. They also need to
build upon the idea of mentoring throughout the educational
experience. For example, faculty should be mentoring students
and mentoring each other in the ways of political activism.

In the public sector, Veronica Stephens recommended that
nurses in appointed positions have the vision to help others and,
in doing so, to mentor their successors. She herself experienced
extremely good mentors who taught her what was expected in the
role she assumed. Stephens expressed concern for the commonly

held opinion that "Nurses eat their young." She feels that we need more time for mentoring, and attributes some of the growth in the Bureau of Prisons to her own mentoring activities. Over time, she has encouraged other nurses to begin the Bureau's training program, and had the vision to build infrastructures so that nursing in the Prison Bureau could grow. Stephens attributes the increase in the number of nurses from 350 to 1,000, and the increase in the number of nurse practitioners from 0 to 50 in part to her own mentoring activities.

LESSON 10: IT TAKES LEARNING ABOUT YOURSELF

Getting politically involved is essential to making change, but choosing what path to take means knowing yourself. While knowing who you are is important before you enter into the political arena, you learn even more about yourself once you are embroiled in the campaign, or hold office or an appointed position. How one handles the joy of winning, the disappointment of losing, the "headiness" of power, or the loss of power, has taught hard lessons to the nurses we interviewed. Each of them has undergone at one time or another the rigors of self-reflection. In the 1970s, at a time of social change for women, Imogene King learned that you have to respect the person first and then the nurse. She learned this lesson in the following way. While serving on the city council, the sign in front of her name initially read "Miss King," while the sign for the dentist who served on the council used the title "Doctor." King confronted the city clerk and asked for the sign to be changed to reflect her credential. In doing this, she made an enemy of the city clerk, but felt she gained respect as a woman and nurse.

Some expressed the personal growth they experienced during the process of running for office or being appointed. Some seemed surprised at the inner strength they exhibited during their campaign. Irma Hart learned the importance of writing skills and took courses in English and basic writing. Margaret Leonard found out that if you work hard enough you, can get what you want. Although she didn't win the election, she was able to win her town. Christine Canavan had to learn what *not* to say. Lois Capps never saw her own leadership potential before her husband died and she decided to run for office. Eve Franklin found out that while everything scares her, nothing stops her. Sharon Cooper learned that her honesty and directness are sometimes a problem. While many noted that men had an easier time asking for money and receiving political support, there seemed to be an optimism or an "I can do it" attitude that prevailed.

Kay Khan began her journey after participating in grassroots activities in her hometown in Massachusetts. She describes how she went about making the decision and taking a chance. She challenged herself to "just do it," and in this instance was successful. Khan explained:

> Approximately 4 to 5 years ago, one of the people I had supported for state legislator stepped down from her office and the community was beginning to look for someone, a pro-choice woman, a candidate from the Democratic party who might be interested in running for office. I thought about it, and had often thought about working up "there" in the state house working on public policy issues. But the thought of actually running for office seemed daunting and that had always held me back. I continued to think about it and began contacting some of the political folks I knew in the city of Newton that I knew were politically savvy, to sort of run it by them and see what they thought about my running. People were enthusiastic, and so I continued to research the possibility— I still felt like I had to get over that threshold of the fear of getting out there and being more visible and being more public and taking that next step, which is to get out there and be very open about what you plan to do.
>
> I subsequently happened to go to a lecture given by a woman psychologist, and she had been invited to come and speak about why women aren't making it to the glass ceiling. What she spoke about was that she had found through the work she had done that women, unlike men, like to know something 200% before they take that next step. And that's the one thing that seems to hold women back. Men are much more apt to jump in and just go for it. After hearing that lecture, I decided that I was definitely in that category. I felt, "What do I know about being a state representative," and so forth. So, I decided to give it a try. What have I got to lose? I began to speak with more people and someone put me in touch with a woman who had run campaigns in the city of Newton. She got very excited and we were off and running. My first campaign began in April of 1994. That was for the election in November of

1994, and my first term began in January of 1995. I am just now beginning my third term. I'll be sworn in tomorrow. It was very interesting, very exciting, a new step for me. I remember saying to my campaign manager, and she reminds me of it every time, I said, "Do we have to do it with bumper stickers and signs?" And she said, "Well, that's the only way for people to get to know you."

Mary Wakefield's story is a bit different. Knowledge about her own interests and beliefs helped her pursue the opportunity to learn about policymaking. She tells the following story:

I was a faculty member at the University of North Dakota in 1987 and I had summers off. I was really interested in health care policies, so I sent a letter to Senator Burdock's office and asked if I could work for him as an unpaid intern or fellow so I could learn about how policies are made at a federal level . . . His office called me and said they had a position open and asked if I had any interest in applying for the job as a legislative assistant. I was clueless as to what I would be getting into because I was never been at that level before . . . but I had always been advocating to my students the importance of their engaging in the policy arena, and as I had mentioned, I had been involved with the state nurses association. So I applied for that position and I got it, and I moved through the ranks pretty quickly.

When Wakefield moved to Washington, an area with a higher cost of living than North Dakota, she took a decrease in her salary. She said she was willing to take that chance because of the opportunity that lay before her.

LESSON 11: IT TAKES FUNDRAISING, FUNDRAISING, AND MORE FUNDRAISING

Almost all of the nurses who ran for public office found fundraising to be one of the most important, yet the most difficult, parts of their campaign. It was easier to fundraise for other candidates and for charities than for oneself. Carolyn McCarthy was fortunate in her fundraising activities during her first campaign. Because of the national attention to the shooting spree on the Long Island Railroad, and her subsequent strong position on gun violence, she received donations from across the United States. Despite this, she admitted that fundraising was the "hardest part" of her job, taking her away from her work as a legislator. She said she appreciated the $5 donations most, because these were the ones that she felt were actually backed by votes.

Some felt that asking for money for a political campaign was difficult because they were women. Christine Canavan felt that people give more money to men than women. She noted that men have an easier time asking for money. Fundraising required a grassroots effort on the part of many. Canavan successfully raised money by holding spaghetti suppers and early morning breakfasts in the community. Several candidates relied on friends, family, and colleagues to finance their campaigns, raising small amounts of money that they used wisely. Running for office meant raising money, and that activity required a lot of attention by the candidate.

In her bid for state senator in New York, Mel Callan received financial support of the Democratic Party. She ran in one of the most expensive state senate campaigns at the time, costing $500,000 to run against her opponent, who spent $600,000. Knowing that it was her responsibility to raise money, she turned to her friends in nursing, her colleagues at work, her family, and community. Her friends in the state nursing association ran "tea bag teas," and East Ridge Family Medicine where she worked as a Nurse Practitioner backed her campaign. Callan lost the first election and ran again soon after. For her second campaign for County Legislature in 1996, she sent letters to donors who had supported her first campaign and received $7,000. While Callan looks at fundraising as a positive experience, she feels that nurses need to become more comfortable with it and encourages nurses to practice this skill by getting involved with the campaigns of others.

Given the crucial nature of fundraising and the powerful influence on the success of an election, Barbara Wright advises that candidates should "just grow up. It's the rules of the road when you are in a democracy!" Wright runs in a competitive district and must fundraise. For the State Assembly race in 1999, she planned to raise $400,000 and proactively sought to do so. In her state, she receives a great deal of support from the party and the Speaker. In fact, they assist in raising money. For the 1999 election, they planned several events intended to capture a wide range of financial supporters. One was held in a ballpark where they charged $250.00 per person, and a less expensive fundraiser was held at the home of a school nurse where the charge was $45.00 per person. Despite the many dollars spent, Wright lost the election by 1,200 votes. Voter turnout (50,000) was low, which may have contributed to the loss. Wright indicated that she may run again in 2001.

State nursing associations served as a source of campaign funds in some instances; however, this kind of support could not always be relied on. Sharon Cooper described her experience of being turned down by her state nursing association. Cooper attributed the lack of support from nursing because of her pro-life stand on abortion. When she spoke before the Georgia Nurses Association, attendees expressed their anger with her politics by booing her. Despite this reaction, Cooper won't close any doors. She feels that nurses need to be more involved and in a way that they can be heard.

While a number of the lessons learned could be viewed as a deterrent to running for office or seeking an appointment to a public position, they should serve as a reality check instead. They are lessons that mimic life, shaping the way people think and act—the winning, the losing, the investing, caring, changing, persevering, affiliating, mentoring, learning, and fundraising—and creating a mindset to pursue political opportunities in service of the public.

REFERENCES

Ashley, J. A. (1973). About power in nursing. *Nursing Outlook, 21*(10), 637–640.

DeParle, J. (1995, November 12). Sheila Burke is the militant feminist commie peacenik who's telling Bob Dole what to think. *New York Times Magazine,* pp. 32–38, 90, 100, 102–104.

Hanley, B. E. (1987). Political participation: How do nurse compare with other professional women? *Nursing Economics, 5,* 179–185.

Maraldo, P. (1985). The illusion of power. In R. R. Wieczorek (Ed.), *Power, politics, and policy in nursing* (pp. 64–73). New York: Springer Publishing Co.

Margolies-Mezvinsky, M. (1994). *A woman's place . . . The freshmen women who changed the face of Congress.* New York: Crown Publishers.

McClure, M. L. (1985). Power in nursing. In R. R. Wieczorek (Ed.), *Power, politics, and policy in nursing* (pp. 55–63). New York: Springer Publishing Co.

Robson, J. B. (1998). One nurse's journey to becoming a policymaker. In D. J. Mason & J. K. Leavitt (Eds.), *Policy and politics in nursing and health care* (3rd ed., pp. 426–435). Philadelphia: Saunders.

Snively, M. A. (1993). Address of President Mary Agnes Snively. In N. Birnbach & S. B. Lewenson (Eds.), *Legacy of leadership: Presidential addresses from the Superintendents' Society and the National League of Nursing Education, 1894–1952* (pp. 34–39). New York: National League for Nursing Press. (Original work published 1898)

Winter, M. K., & Lockhart, J. S. (1997). From motivation to action: understanding nurses' political involvement. *Nursing & Health Care Perspectives, 18*, 244–247.

CHAPTER SIX

Creating Political Opportunities

Nursing, like every form of life activity, is a part of the warp and woof of the whole social fabric. Nursing cannot be an isolated, separated thing-in-itself; the interplay of social forces inevitably as day follows the night exerts an effect on nursing.

—Shirley C. Titus

Throughout this book we have described how nurses have become politically involved and shaped political and health care agendas. They have shared with us how they gravitated toward public service, and they have reflected on their own personal histories and professional growth. While seeking public office, they have learned how to interface with the public and advocate for social change. They have debated, raised money, run for office, won, and lost. Some are legislators or have worked for senators, while others have supported the campaigns of numerous candidates, including family members. They have received blessings and financial backing from their state and national nurses' associations, and a few have been denied the support of organized nursing because of differing political views. Nurses have volunteered on the campaigns of other nursing candidates, organized grassroots support in the community, walked door-to-door to solicit votes, handed campaign materials to early-morning commuters, and attended numerous rallies, meetings, and sports events. They have walked many miles, sent numerous letters and e-mails, appeared on cable television, and spoken at gatherings within their communities. All of these activities have put nursing in the public's eye.

INTERFACE WITH THE PUBLIC

Nurses have always interfaced with individuals, groups, and communities as they went about the business of providing nursing care. In chapter 2, we described the early days of professional nursing and the establishment of the Henry Street Settlement. Of this venture with Mary Brewster, Wald (1915) wrote, "We were to live in the neighborhood as nurses, identify ourselves with it socially, and in brief, contribute to it our citizenship" (pp. 8–9). And so, they interfaced with the public by living within the culture of the Lower East Side. Through this experience they gained the trust of the people who lived in the settlement, provided care, assisted people to learn the necessary resources to maintain a healthy environment, and championed social reform.

This kind of interface is not very different from what we found in the population of nurses who were interviewed. With little exception, they live in the communities they represent through political office, have campaigned and undertaken grassroots efforts in their home communities, and have acted as a resource to the individuals and groups with whom they interact daily. They are also "leading the way" in terms of social reform. The "care" they have provided has been within the context of breaking down barriers and facilitating access to health care, and advocating a healthy, safe environment for people of all ages and backgrounds. Through the many points of interface, these nurses have gained the trust of the public, served as a resource for health-related concerns, and dedicated themselves to what one participant referred to as "caring on a grand scale."

The nurses interviewed for this book have significantly altered the face that the public sees. They have chipped away at the longstanding nursism that has pervaded our society. They have brought issues to the table mirroring the health care concerns of the American public. Given that the public trusts nurses, and that nurses feel a social obligation to meet the public's trust, nurses who serve in appointed or elected positions have a tremendous opportunity to make change.

DEVELOPING PUBLIC TRUST

Interface with the public is obviously greater when there is trust between the parties involved. Being trustworthy means being credible, authentic, and dependable. It means doing what you say and admitting when you can't help or don't have the answers. Capps (1998) said, "This trust makes us the perfect messengers for our families' and communities' health and well-being" (p. 80). In our experience, the educational process that produces nurses supports the notions of authenticity, dependability, responsibility, and accountability. Many of those interviewed spoke about the trust the public has in nurses. The term "credibility" was mentioned frequently, as was "respect." Some spoke of the trust that nurses, as one of their constituent groups, had in them.

There were numerous examples testifying to this high level of trust. One instance came about in the Iowa State Legislature. Beverly Nelson-Forbes told of the following situation:

> Just last week a lady came over to me. The bridge of her nose was full and it was obvious that she had a sinus infection. So she was asking me what she needed to do. And it was kind of interesting because I told her she needed to see her physician. You could see that it was slightly red and so forth. Well, it happened that we had a physician over in the Senate and so she asked somebody else about it and they said "Just go over and see the doctor in the Senate." So she went over and he said it's probably a virus, and you can't take anything for a virus anyhow, and he gave her suggestions for over-the-counter stuff. So she came back [to me] and told me about this. I said, "Well you can do that if you want to, but if it was my head I wouldn't do that." So the next day she went to the clinic and they put her on some allergy medicine plus some antibiotics, and you know she's feeling better.

Because Nelson-Forbes was credible and trusted, the woman accepted her recommendation. While campaigning for the Wisconsin Legislature, Robson (1998) and her "white-shoe army" of nurses reasoned, "It's tough to beat a nurse . . . A nurse running for political office is more than a curiosity (not many run) because we have an intrinsically positive image" (p. 428). Muriel Shore, Carolyn McCarthy, and Paula Hollinger referred to the respect they have experienced and the perception by the public that the agenda they have is not purely political and they are not tied to special interests. Likewise, Eve Franklin said that she is seen as someone who is not always mercenary. Others attested to "having a great rapport with senior citizens," "bridging the distance because of my helper role," and "having clout . . . in addressing some of the issues." Perhaps unique for nurses, trust has been an essential factor in facilitating ascendance to the political arena, enabling the creation of political opportunities that may otherwise not exist.

CREATING POLITICAL OPPORTUNITIES

Nurses have created political opportunities in order to accomplish their personal and professional goals, but with these opportunities come expectations. Kristine Gebbie created opportunities by doing her homework. She had to understand the entity she was serving and the structures that made it work. Gebbie said that "Any chance you have to be at an event with a significant person, take advantage of it. Don't wait for the door to be opened. Do it!" Patricia Montoya said she wanted to share with people, especially minorities, that the opportunities are there. "You can do it. Not everyone comes from families that were oriented that way [raised in a family that is politically oriented]. It is not necessary to follow a structured path." Her background was atypical in the sense that while she was growing up there was no presence or encouragement for Montoya to pursue political activities. Her school health background initially spurred her interest in public service. This interest led her to become involved in her state nurses' association and, subsequently, in the American Nurses Association Office of Political Education. While at ANA, she became known in Washington and received her "political education," in part, by interviewing congressional candidates to gather information for the Office of Political Education (now known as the Political Action Committee of ANA). She also developed grassroots experiences in congressional districts, where she spoke with legislators, the public, and health care professionals about health-related issues. These experiences created the opportunity to be visible to the political "powers that be," that led to appointments as Regional Director of Health and Human Services and then United States Department of Health and Human Services Commissioner for Children, Youth, and Families.

In her book *Taking Back Politics: An Insider's Guide To Winning,* Cathy Allen (1996) said, "Campaigns in the '90s require tremendous amounts of energy (and as much good sense and timing) if they are to succeed" (p. 1). The nurses we interviewed shared this sentiment. Those who ran for office identified the significant amount of time and energy that they expended just in putting their names and faces in front of the public. Each one developed specific strategies that supported election or appointment. Some told us that they approached their campaigns using a people-oriented focus, such as knocking on doors, speaking at public events, or meeting prospective constituents in their homes or places of business. They described using the common-sense approach that their nursing backgrounds taught them and they applied it to winning. Some also recognized that much of what they did was "by the seat of their pants." They learned by their mistakes, and wanted to share their stories with us to help others to avoid the same mistakes.

Allen (1996) wrote her book in order to help candidates who might not fit a typical profile, such as women or minority members, to successfully run political campaigns. She wrote it as a "how-to," with sage advice from campaign consultants, candidates, journalists, pollsters, and others who have supported political campaigns. She said that running for office in the 1990s requires a process that threatens to "overtake the passion" (Allen, 1996, p. 2) of why someone runs for office. Since politics has become a business, Allen explained, good leaders have to be good campaigners. They need to know how to organize their teams, use technology efficiently, listen to the pollsters, use research, find ways to pay for work previously done by volunteers, and be able to transmit their ideas and values to the public.

Allen (1996) gives us some "Golden Rules" for candidates to follow that include:

- There's no one perfect way to run a campaign.
- There are a dozen ways to win.
- No one thing you do will eliminate you.
- Don't try to do everything.
- Beware of meetings.
- Make good business decisions.
- Make sure your chain of command is understood.
- Watch out for your friends.
- Assume nothing.
- Stay informed.

- Focus on what's important.
- Ask everyone for money.
- Never ask a volunteer to do something you wouldn't do yourself (p. 6).

Whether engaged in an election or appointed to a public position, participants gave similar advice. The nurses on the campaign trail or who were appointed learned several of the same skills necessary to compete in an election, sometimes winning over positions held by "inside" candidates. Whether they won or lost, they all wanted not only to share their stories, but also to offer, in a sense, their own set of "golden rules." In this way, they have begun to mentor others who are thinking of following their lead.

ADVICE FROM NURSES INTERVIEWED

Advice was readily given by all participants, and the overwhelming sentiment was to "go for it," to pursue your dreams, and to try to make a difference. The "golden rules" that they cited addressed "how to" get started, become politically aware, present the "right" image, get involved, find support, understand nuance, know that you belong, decide to run, run a campaign, fundraise, have a sense of humor, and seek appointment.

GET STARTED

Whether you plan to run for office or seek a policy-making appointment, or are simply interested in getting politically involved, the advice in this section applies to you. It is important to note that there is no one way to "get started." Many of those interviewed became involved in a variety of ways, for example, some from an abiding sense of what they believed to be right and a commitment to public service, and some because a political issue affected their profession, their practice, or their education. Others felt dissatisfied with the legislative decisionmaking process they saw in government, which rarely sought nursing expertise when addressing health-related legislation. A couple of participants started with a Robert Wood Johnson fellowship that focused on health policy, others through their state or national nurses' associations, and yet others through the military. As she came to know people in Washington, DC, Sheila Burke's friends asked her if she would be interested in working for Senator Robert Dole for a year on his staff. Her work with the senator spanned nearly 20 years. Herschella Horton got involved in her community because she wanted to have input into the county hospital that was being built. As she worked on the campaigns of others, her involvement in politics increased. Others asked her to run, which she did. At the time of our interview, she was the ranking Democrat on the Health Committee of the Arizona House of Representatives. Whatever the reasons for their initial involvement, or whatever ways they began, they all felt compelled to get involved and get started. For many nurses, becoming politically aware is the first step toward running for or holding public office.

BECOME POLITICALLY AWARE

Sage advice given by so many of the nurses interviewed was that organized nursing, and individual nurses, need to know what is going on in the world. To summarize what has already been stated in chapter 5, Mary Wakefield advised nurses:

> to broaden their horizons . . . we can't be speaking nurse speak. One of the things I learned early on is to the extent that I had . . . breadth in topics that I could discuss with people, it really provided an entrée.

Allison Giles also spoke about the need to be "broad-thinking." We need to know the issues in nursing, but we also need to have a global awareness, a sense of how and what we do as nurses fit into the world around us. At the very least, nurses need to read the paper, daily. To counteract the "myopia of nursing," nurses must know what national and local newspapers offer. Additionally, the Internet provides an excellent and expanding source of global information. Knowing the various Internet sites that inform us about world events, as well as about nursing, is essential at this crucial point in history. The media, such as books and newsprint, may become a thing of the past in the 21st century, as new technology presents different ways of disseminating information. For those who are not yet as comfortable with technology as they need to be, getting started could mean learning how to use computers and accessing the Internet.

When getting started, aside from developing global awareness, it is important to be aware of whom you are. Virginia Trotter Betts advised nurses to be in touch with their ideals. Betts became politically active through the professional nursing organization, rather than through a political organization. Ideals, and not party affiliation, helped Betts shape her future in political life. Knowing who you are requires a great deal of self-reflection. Knowing how you relate to others or how you approach problems or how you work on teams is also important, as it allows you to assess your own strengths and shore up any weaknesses. This assessment is essential to "getting started."

PRESENT THE "RIGHT" IMAGE

Andrica (1997) said that nursing "is most strongly perceived by how nurses present themselves. . . . If we feel good about who we are and what we do, we communicate that feeling to others both verbally and nonverbally" (p. 105). She goes on to say that changes in how health care is delivered have enhanced the image of nursing, since they have given nurses an opportunity to have a positive impact on processes and outcomes. Mary Wakefield spoke about how she was perceived by Senator Kent Conrad (D-North Dakota). He introduced her as

> "my chief of staff. She's a nurse, she has her PhD in nursing." I really liked that. As far as I was concerned that wasn't important visibility for me because I was already in that job; but it was important visibility that "Yes, this is something nurses can do and do effectively" and something a United States Senator takes pride in or he wouldn't bother telling his Senate colleagues and others as part of his every introduction.

Participants described the importance of presenting an image that not only supported nursing, but also enhanced the influence of the nurse in public policy. When she entered the Veterans Administration, Nancy Valentine said she was seen as the chief nurse, "with all of the stereotypes attached to the role of nurse." She was hired from outside the VA system. People respected her because she was a novelty, although some were skeptical. In her new role, people see her as "more creative and not as the 'chief nurse.'" She is clear about her nursing identity and promotes nursing. She helped to improve the image of nursing within the organization, which directly benefited the system, e.g., nursing moved from the control of medicine, and 35 chief nurses within the system became vice presidents. As Chief Nurse of the American Red Cross (ARC), Nancy McKelvey has worked to increase the visibility of nursing that was diminished in the mid-'80s when there was a structural change in the ARC. In the new structure, the Nursing and Health Services Department was disbanded, and nurses were incorporated into the various service lines. Thus, visibility of nurses in the field units was lost. McKelvey said that one of her goals is to retrain the field units regarding the value of nurses.

GET INVOLVED

Getting involved in political activity starts at home. Start locally, by learning the interests and culture of the community where you live and know the issues well. You need to find out what goes on in the community and be committed to the issues. Start by identifying the issues and finding answers to some of the concerns in your town.

Pat Latona became involved in politics first as the appointed Traffic Commissioner in her town and later as a candidate for public office. She knew the concerns of her town regarding traffic and the safety issues, so she was able to be part of the solution. She was also Deputy Chairperson of the Planning Board in her town, and in this role she was involved in developing a master plan. This gave her an opportunity to interface with a number of people in her community, for example, lawyers, politicians, architects, and community activists. Allison Giles recommended learning the issues and raising questions about them: "You've got to follow them up, find out how certain decisions were made and if you don't like those decisions [and for her it meant how those decisions would affect her patients], then you have to look at alternatives." To improve a situation means talking about it, participating in campaigns at all levels, and connecting with the right people to make your views known. You cannot focus solely on how the issues will affect your patient alone, but rather how these issues will affect the patient, the community, the economy, or another interested party. So getting involved means considering the many factors in decision making at local, state, and national levels.

Nurses know well how to communicate. They've read books on the subject, heard lectures on therapeutic communication, learned to observe, listen, and be reflective, and practiced the art of negotiation. The verbal and nonverbal skills once learned for use at the bedside hold up rather well in the political arena. Nurses understand the health care needs of people, and once conversant on the issues in a community, they are better able to speak for those who cannot speak for themselves. They become the advocates and champions of those who need support. Herschella Horton advised nurses to think about what they want to do and then get involved. Small accomplishments can be great, and it is important to remember that change does not occur overnight. Horton found that by getting involved, she could be a voice for people who did not have one.

FIND SUPPORT

Public service, whether as a candidate, an elected official, or an appointee, requires support from family, friends, colleagues, organizations, or wherever it is offered. Many of the people we interviewed found that support by family and friends was essential to their success. Without it, they would not have been able to campaign with the same commitment and energy. One daughter of a nurse interviewed flew to her mother's side and ran her campaign. Another candidate, Donna Gentile O'Donnell, said her husband, who had been Speaker of the House in Pennsylvania while he was State Senator, not only helped run the campaign but was her driver, her confidante, and her coach. Christine Canavan's husband appeared with her at many of the political gatherings she attended and was a great "sounding board;" her son also was a tremendous help. Ultimate support came from Judy Uherbelau's daughter. Unbeknownst to Uherbelau, her daughter had an article titled, "Is This a Job Worth Fighting (Fair) For," published in the March 29, 1999 edition of *Newsweek*. The article describes her mother's campaign for state representative and the negative campaigning of her opponent. Fortunately, her mother prevailed with "a

12 percentage-point victory, the largest margin the seat had seen in something like 20 years" (Uherbelau, 1999, p. 14). The nurses who sought public office and public service found support within their family systems. They believed that it was essential and they advised others to develop this kind of support.

Many of the nurses interviewed balanced their lives between husbands, children, work, and public service. They asked their families, friends, and colleagues for their advice when deciding whether or not they should run for public office. When Beverly Nelson-Forbes asked to run for office, she called her five grown children and asked them what they thought. "Oh Mom, that's great," they told her. Even with their support, Nelson-Forbes advised that you need a great committee to help you win the election. She said:

> I think the women work harder to get their husbands elected than the guys do [to get wives elected], which is probably pretty typical. I really had to have a strong committee. I was really by myself. My children didn't live near me and I didn't have any brothers or sisters. My parents are gone, my husband's gone. So I was kind of a lonely chick. I had to have a good committee and primarily have had the same committee for the past three times that I've run. They're tremendous and you've got to have people helping you with events.

Others, such as Joseph Polisena, found great support among their professional colleagues. "They felt like I was one of them," said Polisena. The nurses supported him because of the connection they felt with having a nurse run for state senator.

UNDERSTAND THE NUANCE

Drawing on her many years in politics, Donna Gentile O'Donnell noted:

> Nurses must know that while their nursing skills are transferable to the political arena, they also have to learn a whole new set of skills. You need to learn the territory as well as learn the language of politics. Words and phrases have a different meaning in politics, and you have to learn the "phenomenon of nuance."

O'Donnell likened knowing the political arena and understanding political nuance to riding in a canoe. In her canoe analogy, presented in chapter 3, O'Donnell explained how when canoeing down a river, you need to learn to read the water, to understand the nuance, to go around the rocks and things hidden just below the surface of the water. Similarly, Kristine Gebbie commented on the importance of knowing the structural issues and players to be effective in making change. Shirley Chater also had to learn the "nuance" in relation to expectations about political favors. When directed to find jobs for certain people, so-called political appointments, she needed to defend why she could not make the job placements. Similarly, nurses need to develop the technical skill of politics. For example, people in politics make promises that they don't always keep, and you need the skill to be able read the subtext so that you will know who will or won't keep their promise. You need to be able to read the signposts to guide you through the political waters.

KNOW THAT YOU BELONG

Being an insider in the legislative process is critical to change. Eve Franklin said that there are many levels of government in which to get involved. You need to assess who you are and know what works for you, personally and professionally. If running for a legislative office is not for you, you can get involved in a more conventional way, such as building political networks and establishing community connections. Although her career in politics didn't start until the fifth decade of her life, Barbara Wright spent the preceding years getting ready. She was a childbirth educator when New Jersey moved toward family-centered nursing care, chairperson of the New Jersey State Nurses Association's committee to change the definition of nursing in New Jersey, Executive Director of the New Jersey State Nurses Association where she had a professional role in shaping public policy, Mayor of Plainsboro, and then Assemblywoman. She said she often had an understanding of the issues that others did not. She is acutely aware of her unique position, having said, "I'm in as powerful a position as I can be, given the time in office and the fact that I'm a woman."

Nursing builds self-confidence, and it is that self-confidence and trust that assure a sense of belonging and a rightful place at the table. Although no nurse has ever held a seat in the United

States Senate, Eddie Bernice Johnson expressed the need for such a combination. Not withstanding the high cost of running such a race and the high need for name recognition, Johnson felt it was possible for a nurse to run for senator. To be successful in such a race, Johnson advised running in one of the smaller states, where you don't need millions of dollars for the campaign and there are fewer "media markets" that require money. Johnson noted that she spends most of her time working on campaign issues and not on media-seeking.

DECIDE TO RUN

When deciding to run, Imogene King suggests getting together with people who have run campaigns to find out what it's all about. She said, "Decide why do you want to run for office, what do you want to bring, what do you want to do, and what kind of decisions should be made that are not being made." You need to know this because you will be giving a lot of time and energy to the campaign and office if you are really committed. Most of the people we interviewed said, "Just do it!" Christine Canavan said, "Don't worry about whether you'll win or lose, just do it." Name recognition is important to a successful campaign, and many win the second and third time out. Feeling that you do not have the name recognition, while important, should not keep you from running. The more you put your name before the public, the more likely it is that you will be known and have credibility, improving the chances of winning the next time. Eileen Cody also urged nurses to "Do it!" To assuage the fear of feeling that you don't know enough or the overwhelming idea of running for office, Cody advised nurses that they are really well prepared for this role: "You don't have to be an expert at first, nor is running for office as intimidating as it seems."

Several people said that you need a thick skin in politics, but they noted that you need that in nursing as well. Nurses have practice in "being thick-skinned." They have had to deal with hospital administrators, community boards, physicians, patients, and each other. They have had to navigate the politically charged waters of hospitals, home care, and university settings. Politics is not new to nurses. We have had to be political since the modern nursing movement began in the 1870s and even before that! You

just have to decide if you can transfer this aptitude into a political career. More importantly, you need to know when you are in
the right place at the right time to take advantage of opportunities
that come along. Knowing the political culture of your community
is another way of learning to "read the water." Eve Franklin called
for the use of a systematic approach to your life work, finding a
balance between the many roles you undertake such as a nurse,
legislator, family member, or appointee. Franklin advised that
you must learn to "balance altruism with pragmatism" to survive
and be effective.

RUN A CAMPAIGN

Most advice columns for campaigns stress the need to find a
good campaign manager. Kay Khan also supports this notion,
emphasizing that the campaign manager is extremely important
to the success of a candidacy. The campaign manager can organize the many facets of the campaign and allow the candidate to
focus on the issues. Even with a great campaign manager, first
campaigns can be the hardest. Khan described her own as "the
toughest." Here she presents her story:

> My first campaign was the toughest. I had five men running against
> me. I would say four of the men and myself were all pretty much
> the same on the issues. We were all fairly progressive liberal
> Democrats and Newton is a progressive Democratic city. I had to
> distinguish myself in some way other than just being the only
> woman. I think that [being a nurse] definitely helped. I think that
> my health care background and pushing that was also key, and peo-
> ple were very interested in that. Two of the men that I ran against
> were actually long-term members of the local Board of Aldermen.
>   I knew it was going to be an uphill battle because of their name
> recognition. But I think that I had much more name recognition
> than those folks realized. I had lived in the community, at that
> point, for 24 years. I raised three children in the city of Newton
> who had attended the Newton public schools. My activities with
> the Newton Democratic City committee and my membership at
> the local hospital as a staff person . . . all of those things came
> together to be very helpful in the end.
>   I had to raise money. I organized a campaign committee. I was
> very fortunate in having a fundraiser in the beginning of my first
> campaign in which I did extremely well and was able to raise about

$20,000 with one campaign party. And that really got me off the ground and running. I really had a lot of support. Again, I think raising that kind of money, because women generally have a harder time raising money, and having a health care background were the two things that were instrumental in sending me over the top.

I did very well in subsequent campaigns—interestingly, in the first campaign, I won in the end in the final. I had a primary and then I had a final. In the end I won by 71% and I really thought that I wouldn't have opposition the second time out. [Then] I did not have a primary; [but] I did have a final. And I won by 76% and yet again someone came out, a Republican, a woman who gave me a good run for my money. But I did win. This time, by 72%. With a lot of hard work, we did raise quite a bit of money again. So I think the first campaign I raised about $45,000 and spent it all. The second, I raised about $25,000 and spent it all; and this one, close to $35,000 and spent it all. It's very expensive because of the cost of stamps and brochures and mailings, etc.

Running a campaign means knowing how to delegate to others and trusting the chaos that will ensue. Rolling with the punches, and being flexible and able to work with others, are among the skills that one needs to run a successful campaign. Being a realist while keeping a positive attitude takes fortitude, and courage is also important.

LEARN TO FUNDRAISE

Campaigns need money. Money pays for telephones, "volunteers," mailings, posters, fliers, meetings, food, supplies, rent, overhead, advertisement, media coverage, babysitters, and so forth. The list is endless regarding the amount of money needed to get your name and face out there before the public. In order to run for office, you need to fundraise. Yet, fundraising seemed to be the one area that those interviewed found the most difficult and most challenging. Paula Hollinger noted that newcomers to campaigns find fundraising difficult. People, she said, prefer to give their money to candidates they have heard of, rather than to a newcomer, especially a female candidate. In the previous section, Khan noted that women usually have more difficulty raising money. Most of the people we interviewed said that they were uncomfortable about asking for money for themselves. They had less trouble when it was for someone else.

Given the importance of fundraising, the nurses interviewed said that you have to learn this skill. Having mounted a successful $500,000 state senate campaign, Mel Callan challenged nurses to become more comfortable with fundraising, saying that nurses needed to practice this skill by working on the campaigns of others. Callan looked at fundraising as a positive experience and encouraged others to fundraise for a nurse colleague. In this way, you learn the skill and support someone who shares similar professional goals and values. A few people referred to EMILY (Early Money Is Like Yeast) and EMILY's List, an organization that one person indicated has supported "every nurse who has run for office," as a source to help with fundraising. One way to get started with fundraising is to give money to a campaign. In this way, we begin the practice of supporting candidates and prepare ourselves to ask others to contribute.

HAVE A SENSE OF HUMOR

In running a campaign, aside from the need for a great campaign manager and to be adept at fundraising, you need to set priorities, you need to be decisive, and, perhaps most important, you need a sense of humor. While campaigns have a limited time-frame, they can take on a life of their own, and so you have to be able to distinguish yourself from the others and be able to survive the strong (and sometimes negative) competition you will face. A sense of humor will help you survive the winning and the losing as well as the job itself.

Another side to this is learning not to take yourself too seriously. An example of this comes from Paula Hollinger, whose campaign materials and strategies lent humor to her campaign. She rewrote the words to a popular 1960s song, "Hey, Hey, Paula":

Hey, Hey, Paula
I want to vote for you
Hey, Hey, Paula
No one else could ever do

You fought for more jobs
and improved health care, too
Hey, Hey, Paula. . . . [then there is some spoken dialogue about her record of accomplishments, and the refrain is repeated at the end]

For 2 weeks of radio campaigning, the rewritten song was sung. Hollinger said that people were "singing the tune all over." One of her campaign brochures says, "This nurse makes house calls," and another has a picture of Frankenstein's monster to convey the "monster" of high taxes. The latter brochure reads, "It was a monster . . . A $554,000 Tax Monster! In fact, it was the largest tax increase in Maryland history . . . and Janice Piccinini was the only Baltimore County Senator to vote for it."

SEEK APPOINTMENT

Seeking an appointment to a public office requires no less commitment, skill, or drive than running for office. One must be passionate, persistent, and persuasive in order to be successful. Exercising these essential political skills will help get your ideas across to those who hold the power to appoint. Decide on which issues you want to promote, and focus on two or three objectives. Your ability to persuade and convince others of the relevance and importance of these objectives will determine the nature of the outcomes.

There are a number of strategies that have been used to seek out and/or be sought for political appointments. Mary Moseley assertively "showed up" in the offices of Senator Bill Frist and talked her way to a "yes" when appointed to his staff. Sheila Burke was asked by a friend to consider a staff appointment with Senator Robert Dole. Virginia Trotter Betts applied through a paid fellowship and became a health legislative assistant to Senator Al Gore. According to Carolyne Davis (Berkowitz, 1995), she was appointed as HCFA (Health Care Financing Administration) Administrator by a somewhat circuitous route. She had been Dean, then Associate Vice President for Academic Affairs at the University of Michigan, Ann Arbor in the 1970s. During this time she became interested in federal capitation and NIH grants programs, and reached out to legislators in her state on behalf of her university. This led to a close relationship with Congressman Dave Stockman, for whom she later testified against President Jimmy Carter's proposed program of cost controls. Stockman eventually became the head of the Office of Management and Budget. Their relationship led her to meet other congressional leaders and be considered for the HFCA position.

For many seeking a political appointment or governmental policymaking position, maintaining a bipartisan stance served them well. Shirley Chater felt her nursing background, rather than her political affiliation as an independent, was more important to her appointment by Democratic President Bill Clinton. Had she been a Republican, however, she said that she might have not been appointed. On the other hand, Donna Gentile O'Donnell clearly identified herself as a Democrat and had supported many Democratic candidates before running for office and then being appointed as Deputy Commissioner of Health in the city of Philadelphia. O'Donnell noted, however, that while she has definite party leanings, nurses must recognize the utility of being bipartisan.

LESSONS LEARNED: PARTING WORDS

The nurses we interviewed provided stories of their ventures into political life. While these were never easy, these nurses have forged new ground for others who want to expand their nursing into the public sector. They came into political life from various backgrounds, but each came with a commitment to give back and do something for others. They have made significant changes in legislation affecting health care throughout the many parts of the country, and they continue to advocate improvement in the health care system. These nurses support the profession and most have been supported in kind. Lessons learned have been shared with us and their advice will serve others in the future. Parting words included: "Be action-oriented, come with some kind of solution to the problem"; "Find out what goes on in your community"; "Establish early money"; and "Stay connected with your roots." Beth Mazzella said,

> At times I am the only female, sometimes the only health care professional with a traditional degree, and at times the only nurse in a room. When you are trying to advance your position in some of these places, that is the only tool that you have. When do you take the tool out of the toolbox? If the only tool you have is a hammer, then the only thing that you use is a hammer and the only thing you see is a nail. We have lots of screws and bolts and everything else out there that we have to deal with.

Carolyn McCarthy advised, "Hold your representatives and senators responsible for their actions. It's a privilege to be able to do so.

Don't waste it." Janegale Boyd said that nurses need to provide legislators with data and knowledge. This was echoed by Patricia Montoya, who, as leader of a non-profit organization to recruit nurses to rural areas, came to be seen as a rural health expert when she lobbied legislators to gain support for this organization.

ADVICE TO PREPARE NURSES OF THE FUTURE

Some final thoughts and advice on what we have learned from this experience can be related to what has to happen in the future. There are still too few health care professionals, particularly nurses, in policymaking positions, whether they are elected or appointed. We all need to become involved in some way in order to make changes in our health care system and the lives of the people in our communities that we, as professionals, know should occur. Andrica (1997) asks, "So how can nursing contribute to these changes? First, no one can do it for us. We must take the risks and inspire others" (p. 105). In helping to prepare the nurse of the future to take risks and inspire others, lead the way in policy development and legislation, and advance the public face of nursing, we reflect here on what needs to be done in education, research, and practice.

EDUCATE POLITICALLY MINDED NURSES

Knowing how important their nursing education was to their development as politically active professionals, participants advised integrating political activism throughout undergraduate and graduate nursing curricula. Nursing students at all levels should be engaged in campaigns. Making participation in a political campaign a course or program requirement, or having students take a practicum with someone who is in an elected or appointed position, are two ways to involve them in politics early in the their professional life. Giving students credit for fulfilling a school requirement both lends credibility to political activism and underscores its importance and the responsibility of nurses to be involved. Nursing educators must approach political activism as a nursing role that needs to be taught and nurtured.

Only a few of the nurses we interviewed served on nursing faculties, yet many gave us wonderful ideas about ways to teach students about political activism. For example, faculty can mentor students by bringing them to meetings of professional organization and community action groups. Each course can include a political element in the content, and assignments can reflect this. Other assignments, such as reading the newspaper, monitoring the Internet for health care legislation, attending town meetings, working on campaigns, lobbying Congress, writing letters to public officials, organizing letter writing campaigns, fundraising, writing letters to the editor, or supporting candidates are examples of how assignments can support political activity content. Bringing into class nurses who are involved in political action or who are appointed or elected to public positions exposes students to role models, which can have a far greater impact on students than simply telling them about involved nurses.

Given that faculty serve as role models and mentors to students they, too, need to demonstrate their understanding of and participation in political activity. As with students, faculty need to be involved. For example, New York State Nurses Association (NYSNA) offers a legislative day and other activities designed to prepare students, faculty, and practitioners to become politically active citizens. In a course on health care policy given at Pace University, New York, successful class assignments have involved sending undergraduate and graduate students to lobby at the state capital. Faculty and students have attended Lobby Day together, allowing for the interchange of ideas and modeling behaviors. During one semester, one student served as a role model for the rest of the class and the faculty by actively lobbying a change in the law about the first assistant in the operating room. She scheduled meetings with her peers, prepared written documentation with the talking points they needed to use, arranged appointments with legislators, and presented her activities in class in lieu of another assigned paper. Another class held formal presentations at city hall to inform policy makers about the ins and outs of drug abuse. This was done at a time when there was a great deal of debate about the city's position on treatment programs.

When teaching a course, such as community health or health care policy, using the local and national newspapers as "texts" can be extremely valuable. Also, reading the magazines that the lay public read allows students to keep abreast of current events and get a feel for what people in the community are reading. Faculty need to know how to use the newspaper and how to track a story about a particular bill or health-related concern. They need to be aware that students may need help in understanding how keeping current with social issues applies to the nursing role. One student in a master's course on health care policy incredulously asked when she was assigned the newspaper to read, "Do you really want me to read a paper everyday?" The class was also aghast when the answer was, "Yes." In a class on decision making, students were asked at the beginning of the semester to follow a news story about a developing problem with mosquito-borne encephalitis in a major region of the country. Since faculty did not know how the story would "end," they were able to suspend their own "control" of information to study, along with the students, the issue of spraying insecticide in the community. The topic was discussed later in the semester, and the political issues were dealt with at that time.

Nursing curricula at all levels must include the use of technology to prepare the practitioners of today and the future. It is imperative that we include technology as one source of information and communication; at this point, it almost borders on unethical practice if we do not. Students must be able to write, review the literature and the news, and share information on computers. They must be prepared to use the Internet and access it regularly as a source of information. Students can also "chat" with other people around the world about issues affecting health care. Online browsing should be encouraged and assignments should reflect a global awareness and relevance to their work as nursing professionals. Understanding and using technology are essential steps in preparing politically aware nurses for the future.

RESEARCH TO INFORM AND GUIDE

One of the major lessons learned in writing this book relates to how little is known of nursing's political activism throughout its history. The nursing literature about health and public policy and political activism that does exist offers few articles describing research devoted to the subject. Nursing research can provide

insight about who runs for office, describe what traits are needed to get involved, chronicle who has run and who has been
appointed in the past, and explain why nurses get involved and
why they don't. Both qualitative and quantitative studies are
needed to fully understand these and other questions. For example, in qualitative studies, the use of phenomenology to explore
the lived experiences of politically active nurses would add to
the literature. Historical studies to explicate past political
involvement by nurses may help us understand the factors that
have influenced the untoward image of nurses as apolitical or
subservient.

While we know that many nurses have served in appointed
governmental positions, especially during periods of war, little is
known about these women and the effect they may have had on
decision-making and policy development. Nurses whose backgrounds and experiences could be highlighted include Florence
Blanchfield, who served during World War II as the Superintendent
of the Army Nurse Corps; Sue S. Dauser, who served as Superintendent of the Navy Nurse Corps; and Lucille Petry Leone, who
served as the administrator of the United States Cadet Nurse
Corps and, later, as the Assistant Surgeon General of the United
State Public Health Service. The stories of these women need to
be told and shared with both nurses and the public. As well, it
would be important to use historical research methods to uncover the names of other nurses who have served in public office
and begin to analyze the strategies they used.

Collecting quantitative data on nurses who have run for public
office, whether or not they have won, lost, or been appointed,
has been difficult. Smaller, more community-based studies need
to be conducted to ascertain the numbers and types of candidates in specific geographic areas, as well as nationally. Learning
who these women and men are, how they are perceived by the
public, how they became politically active, how their own personal and professional history affected their political activism,
and the impact they have made are important to understand so
that greater numbers of nurses may follow suit. We can study
nursism and the affect of such prejudice on who enters the profession and how the profession is viewed. Overcoming the effects
of nursism, something that the nurses we interviewed accomplished, would be important to study and understand. For example,

what are the qualities of the individuals who are able to over-come the prejudice of nursism and take on leadership roles in the public arena?

Many of the nurses we interviewed felt they could not do their jobs without data about the issues. They knew how important it was for them to know the research on the topics they addressed in order to intelligently debate their point and effectively make change. In light of the overall data scarcity, we will not fully understand the issues, nor the attempts, successes, and failures that nurses have made in the political arena. Lack of a research base also influences how we approach the future. It is key that we establish programs of research as soon as possible to gather baseline and subsequent data, so that we may plan, implement, and evaluate approaches and decisions in regard to public and health policy initiatives.

PRACTICE INFORMS POLITICAL ACTION

One of the people we interviewed said that the hardest group to convince why she was politically involved was other nurses in practice. Many did not "get it." Many did not see how her running for office or holding a political appointment affected the health of patients. Nurses in practice know the issues. They work with them everyday. They know the regulations and limitations of their nurse practice act, and they see how the health mainte-nance organizations and managed care delivery systems limit the kind of care that they give and that their patients are "entitled" to receive. An excellent example of how this knowledge was effec-tively used to inform the populace at large was described in the September 1999 edition of *Report*, the official newsletter of the New York State Nurses Association ("Montefiore nurse," 1999). This news story told of the July 23, 1999 airing of the "News Hour with Jim Lehrer," a nationally televised program, where a nurse, Judy Sheridan-Gonzalez, "single-handedly punctured" the argu-ments of physicians who supported managed care. She used her practice as a basis for her remarks. She said, "Managed care gives you incentive to undertreat your patients. Managed-care organi-zations put pressure on hospitals to reduce costs. That trans-lates into fewer staff dealing with more patients, who have more complicated problems and go home sicker" (Montefiore nurse,

1999, p. 16). These remarks were a segue to her "plea for whistle-blower protection for healthcare workers . . . [that would enable nurses] to let the public know about the abuses and excesses in the system" (Montefiore nurse, 1999, p. 16). Whistle-blower legislation was a controversial and significant political football that dominated many local, state, and national health care legislative discussions in the late 1990s.

Using the knowledge of practitioners to its best advantage means that nurses must participate in their professional organizations, become aware of their own value and worth, and be encouraged to be active in shaping the political agenda. Nurses can give testimony, write letters, lobby for change, work on campaigns, send money to candidates of their choice, vote, get others to vote, and be aware of the issues. As health care providers, nurses are trusted members of society. They need to value their knowledge and be able to articulate their ideas in political forums. If the voices of nurses "are not represented at the policy table . . . the policies that result will be driven by the dominant values of the public sphere that have left many of our communities struggling for survival" (Backer, Costello-Nikitas, Mason, McBride, & Vance, 1993, p. 75).

So many of those we interviewed felt that their nursing practice provided the depth and breadth they needed on issues that came before legislative bodies. Whether they practiced in acute care settings or community health sites, they found themselves better informed by their work as nurses. One nurse said that she knew what families needed; she had worked with them for over 20 years. Others noted that their nursing practice made them pragmatic. Many continued to practice as they served their terms in state congresses. This gave them both credibility and visibility with the public. Their work in public office was informed by their nursing practice. Nurses who practice need to know this and need to get politically involved. It is part of their practice. Continuing education programs on political activism can also serve as a way to get nurses started and to be more reflective and global in their perspective.

The public face of nursing needs to be exposed and recognized in order for nurses to be able to feel that they have participated and fulfilled their civic responsibility and social commitment to the public. We believe this book has contributed to the process. It is just a beginning.

REFERENCES

Allen, C. (1996). *Taking back politics: An insider's guide to winning.* Seattle, WA : Jalapeno Press.

Andrica, D. (1997, April). Nursing image: Our public relations responsibility. *Nursing Economic$, 15*(2), 105.

Backer, B. A., Costello-Nikitas, D., Mason, D. J., McBride, A. B., & Vance, C. (1993). Power at the policy table: When women and nurses are involved. *Revolution: The Journal of Nurse Empowerment, 3,* 68–76.

Berkowitz, E. (1995). HCFA oral history interview: Interview of Carolyne Davis in her office in Washington, DC, on 8 November 1995. Available online: http://www.ssa.gov/search97cgi

Capps, L. (1998, September). Nurses' voices needed in halls of Congress. *American Journal of Nursing, 98*(9), 80.

Montefiore nurse gives 'em hell: "Jim Lehrer News Hour" viewers get the truth about managed care. (1999, September). *Report, 30*(8), 16.

Robson, J. B. (1998). One nurse's journey to becoming a policymaker. In D. J. Mason & J. K. Leavitt (Eds.), *Policy and politics in nursing and health care* (3rd ed., pp. 426–435). Philadelphia: Saunders.

Titus, S. C. (1991). The new Scutari. In N. Birnbach & S. Lewenson (Eds.), *First words: Selected addresses from the National League for Nursing 1894–1933* (pp. 344–353). New York: National League for Nursing Press. (Original work published 1933)

Uherbelau, A. (1999, March 29). My turn: Is this a job worth fighting (fair) for? *Newsweek,* p. 14.

Wald, L. D. (1915). *The house on Henry Street.* New York: Henry Holt & Company.

Individuals Interviewed for This Book*

Virginia Trotter Betts, MSN, JD, RN, FAAN
Senior Advisor on Nursing and Policy to the Secretary and Assistant
   Secretary of Health
Department of Health and Human Services
Washington, DC

Sheila P. Burke, RN, MPA, FAAN
Executive Dean and Lecturer in Public Policy
Harvard University
John F. Kennedy School of Government

Mary Eileen (Mel) Callan, RN, MS, CS-FNP
Nurse Practitioner
Rochester, New York

The Honorable Christine E. Canavan, BSN
Democratic Massachusetts State Legislator

The Honorable Lois Capps
United States House of Representatives
California, 22nd District

The Honorable Shirley S. Chater
Former Commissioner, United States Social Security Administration
   (1993–1997)
Visiting Professor, University of California at San Francisco,
   Institute for Health and Aging, School of Nursing

---

* Names listed as requested at the time of the interview.

Washington State Representative Eileen L. Cody, RN
11th District

Representative Sharon Cooper
Georgia State Representative

Representative Cindy Empson
Republican Kansas State Representative
District 12

State Senator Eve Franklin, MSN, RN
Great Falls, Montana

Kristine M. Gebbie, DrPH, RN, FAAN
Former National AIDS Policy Coordinator, The White House
Elizabeth Standish Gill Associate Professor of Nursing and Director,
　Center for Health Policy, Columbia University School of Nursing,
　New York

Allison Giles
Legislative Strategies
Washington, DC

The Honorable Marilyn Goldwater
Maryland State Legislator

Irma R. (Sam) Hart, RN
National Manager
Health Awareness Program Federal Aviation Administration
Washington, DC

Paula Colodny Hollinger
Maryland State Senator (D)
District in Baltimore County

Herschella Horton
Assistant Democratic Leader
Arizona House of Representatives

Eddie Bernice Johnson
Member of Congress
United States Representative
District 30, Texas

Representative Kay Khan
Newton, Massachusetts

Imogene King, RN, EdD, FAAN
Former Alderman, Wood Dale, Illinois
Professor Emeritus
University of South Florida in Tampa

Patricia Latona
Director for the Center for Continuing Education in Nursing,
    Distance Learning, and International Programs
Division of Nursing
New York University, New York

Marilyn B. Lee
Hawaii State Representative
38th District

Margaret Leonard
Vice President of Clinical Services
HealthSource, New York

Kate Malliarakis, RN, CNP, MSM, NCADC II
Branch Chief of Specific Drugs
Executive Office of the President/Office of National Drug
    Control Policy
Washington, DC

Rear Admiral Beth Mazzella
Assistant Surgeon General
United States Public Health Service
Office of the Chief Nurse

Representative Mary McGrattan
Connecticut State Legislator

The Honorable Carolyn McCarthy
4th Congressional District
Long Island, New York

Nancy S. McKelvey, MSN
Chief Nurse
American Red Cross

Patricia Montoya, RN, MPA
Commissioner for Children, Youth, and Families
United States Department of Health and Human Services
Washington, DC

Beverly Nelson-Forbes, PhD
Iowa State House of Representatives

LTC Rosemary Nelson
Program Manager and Chief Information Officer
Pacific Region Program Office
Tripler Army Medical Center

Maureen O'Connell
Republican Assembly Member
17th District
Nassau County, New York

Donna Gentile O'Donnell
Deputy Commissioner of Health for Policy and Planning
City of Philadelphia

Joseph M. Polisena, RN, MEd
Former Senator, State of Rhode Island
District #28, Johnston, Rhode Island

Susan Reinhard
Deputy Commissioner of the Department
New Jersey Department of Health and Senior Services

Judy Iris Biros Robson, RN, MSN
Democratic Senator
Wisconsin

Bonnie Ryan
Chief
Veterans Administration Home and Community-Based Care

Claire Shulman
President, Borough of Queens
Queens, New York

Muriel Shore, EdD, CNAA
Mayor
Fairfield, New Jersey

Mary Jane Simmons
State Representative
Massachusetts

Capt. Veronica Stephens
Nurse Practitioner
Former Chief Nurse
United States Bureau of Prisons

Dr. Mary Tennies-Moseley
Formerly of the Office of Senator Bill Frist
Tennessee

Representative Judy Uherbelau
Oregon State Representative

Representative Patricia Vance
Pennsylvania State Representative

Nancy Valentine
Special Assistant to the Under Secretary for Health
United States Department of Veterans Affairs

Mary Wakefield, PhD, RN, FAAN
Professor and Director, Center for Health Policy and Ethics
George Mason University, Virginia
Member, Medicare Payment Advisory Commission (MedPAC)

The Honorable Barbara W. Wright, PhD, RN
Assemblywoman, District 14
New Jersey

Political Action Databases and Audiovisuals on Nurses and Politics

POLITICAL ACTION DATABASES

http://ciir2.cs.umass.edu/Govbot/—A database containing over 1,594,012 Web pages related to the U.S. government.

http://www.ezgov.com/portal/index.jsp—Allows for location of public leaders and services based on zip codes.

http://www.dhhs.gov/—The Department of Health and Human Services Website, which allows for searches of the Office of the Secretary's Web pages. This site also allows you to browse in the Organizational Directory, search the Employee Directory, and search the Health and Human Services Agency for page links.

http://www.gksoft.com/govt/en/us.html—Comprehensive database of governmental institutions on the World Wide Web: parliaments, ministries, offices, law courts, embassies, city councils, public broadcasting corporations, central banks, multigovernmental institutions, etc.

http://www.ana.org/—American Nurses Association Website, which provides access to searches, direct links to affiliate organizations, and legislative updates.

http://www.nursingworld.org./index.htm—Nursing World, a division of the ANA Website.

http://www.nurseweek.com/—Nurseweek/Healthweek Online provides news articles, legislative updates, and links to related Websites, which include: search engines, government, hospitals, and news groups.

http://www.op.nysed.gov/home.html—Office of the Professions for New York State Website with links to its news page and to New York State's Educational Department homepage.

http://www.nysna.org/—New York State Nurses Association Website provides links to issues regarding legislation, practice, nursing, education, news, and other search engines.

http://www.osha.gov/—Occupational Safety and Health Organization Website provides free access to its online journal and links to the Department of Labor, libraries, regulations, and search engines.

http://www.midwife.org—American College of Nurse-Midwives Website offers a site search, web resources, Congressional links, and professional information.

http://www.geocities.com/HotSprings/9483—Midwives Alliance of New York offers updates from state and national midwifery groups, the politics of midwifery and homebirth in New York State, and consumer action.

http://www.mana.org—Midwives Alliance of North America Webpage has links to MANA information, press information, conferences, regional information, and related organizational and international contacts.

http://www.aanp.org—American Academy of Nurse Practitioners provides links related to its foundation, its action hotline, conferences, the 200 elections, healthcare sites, healthcare industry information, legislation, practice information, regulatory information, and searches.

http://www.nurse.org/acnp—American College of Nurse Practitioners Website provides links to Medicare, Medicaid, legislation, affiliates, news, symposiums, searches, and more.

http://www.nysconp.org—New York State Coalition of Nurse Practitioners provides links for its overview, government affairs, and leadership directories.

http://www.nln.org—National League for Nursing Website provides access to online journal and media, trends in nursing education, states leagues information, and search engines.

AUDIOVISUALS ON NURSES IN POLITICS

A case study in shaping health care policy: The National Center for Nursing Research. (1996). New York: National League for Nursing.

Grassroots lobbying: A great tool for nurses. (1991). Washington, DC: American Nurses Association.

Key concepts in public policy. (1986). New York: National League for Nursing.

Nurse power through legislative action. (1993). Guilderland, NY: New York State Nurses Association.

Nurses making a difference: Politics in action. (1998). Washington, DC: American Nurses Association.

Nurses and politics: Shaping the future. (1989). Kansas City, MO: American Nurses Association.

Nursing in America: A history of social reform. (1993). New York: National League for Nursing.

Nursing in America: Through a feminist lens. (1993). New York: National League for Nursing.

The power of nursing. (1993). New York: National League for Nursing.

RNs advocating for patients and nurses: The nurse practice act and the legislative process. (1998). Latham, NY: New York State Nurses Association.

Campaign Posters and Photographs

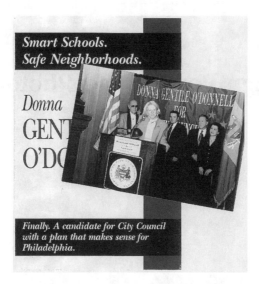

Campaign materials reprinted courtesy of Deputy Commissioner Donna Gentile O'Donnell (also pictured is Nursing Dean Emeritus Claire Fagin).

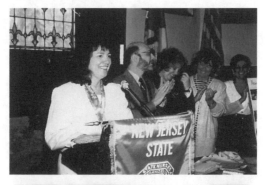

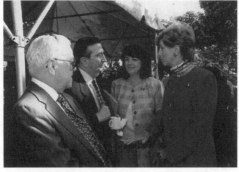

Campaign materials reprinted courtesy of Deputy Commissioner Susan Reinhard.

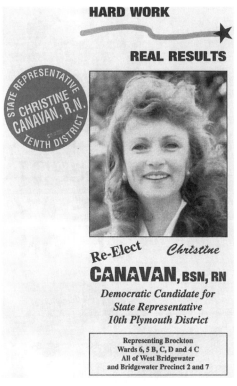

Reprinted courtesy of The Honorable Christine E. Canavan, BSN, RN.

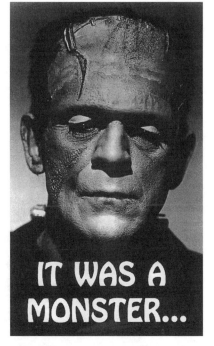

("It" refers to taxes.) Campaign materials reprinted courtesy of Paula Hollinger, Maryland State Senator.

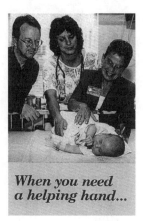

Campaign materials reprinted courtesy of Paula Hollinger, Maryland State Senator.

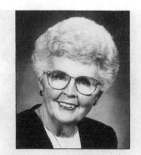

RE-ELECT
BEVERLY
NELSON

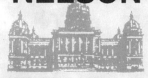

FOR EFFECTIVE REPRESENTATION
IOWA HOUSE DISTRICT 64

Campaign materials reprinted courtesy of Beverly Nelson, Iowa State Representative.

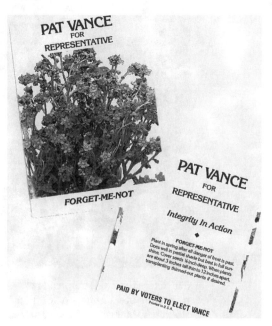

Campaign materials reprinted courtesy of Patricia Vance, Pennsylvania State Representative.

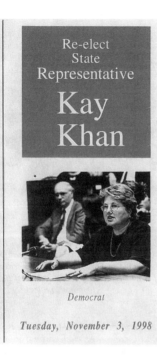

Campaign materials reprinted courtesy of Kay Khan, Massachusetts State Representative.

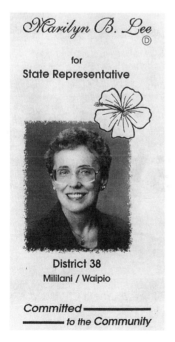

Campaign materials reprinted courtesy of Marilyn Lee, Hawaii State Representative.

August, 1992

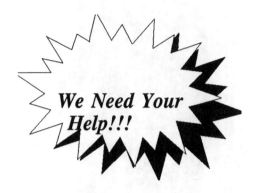

Dear Colleague:

Allow us to bring to your attention a nursing colleague and neighbor of ours who probably does not need any introduction. Muriel Shore, EdD, RN, CNAA, has played a very active role in the nursing field for over 20 years. Muriel was recently re-elected to a 2nd term on the Board of Directors of the American Nurses Association, is a member of the New Jersey State Board of Nursing and is past President of the New Jersey State Nurses Association. Muriel has also been an activist for nursing issues both nationally and in the states of New Jersey and New York.

Dr. Shore now has the opportunity to run for City Council in our home town of Fairfield. She needs your support to achieve what we hope will be just the first step in a political career. As nurses who live in Fairfield, we are actively working to have Muriel elected. We are all extremely excited at the idea of a committed Nurse being an advocate of the people and bringing "Nursing Issues" into the mainstream of politics.

As colleagues and friends of Muriel, we are asking you to join our efforts by contributing to her campaign fund. All donations large or small will be appreciated.

Sincerely,

Kathleen C. Wendowski, MS, RN, LNHA - Ruth Regan Hutchison, DPh, R

Name_____

My donation for Muriel Shore, EdD, RN, CNAA

    $10_____$20_____$50_____$100_

    Please make check payable to Nurses to El
    return to:
                    158 Sand Road
                    Fairfield, NJ 07004

Campaign materials reprinted courtesy of Muriel Shore, Fairfield City Mayor.

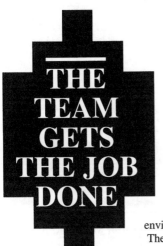

THE TEAM GETS THE JOB DONE

Vote THE TEAM for your security and our children's future.

During the years **Senator Ruth Solomon** and **Representatives Herschella Horton** and **Marion Pickens** have served in the Arizona Legislature, they worked together as a team.

They sponsored legislation to improve neighborhood schools, and they made sure that day-care centers will continue to be safe for our children. Because of THE TEAM's efforts, criminal environmental polluters can still be prosecuted.

They co-sponsored legislation to bring our share of tax dollars to Pima County, and co-sponsored legislation to reduce business inventory taxes.

Solomon, Horton and Pickens safeguarded your rights and the needs of our children. They balanced the need for economic development and

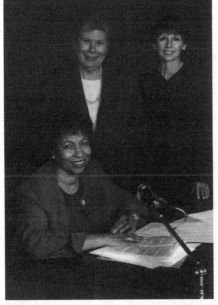

the creation of new jobs with environmental protection. They did this together through their strong leadership, experience, knowledge and plain hard work.

Because of their fight to keep neighborhood streets safe, THE TEAM has won the endorsement of Arizona's Fraternal Order of Police and the state's firefighters.

Vote for Legislators *WHO GET THE JOB DONE.*

There's much more to do.

VOTE THE TEAM

November 5

Campaign materials reprinted courtesy of Herschella Horton (seated), Arizona State Representative.

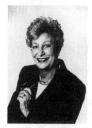

MARILYN GOLDWATER
for
HOUSE OF DELEGATES
District 16

**LEADERSHIP
EFFECTIVENESS
VISION**

A friend Maryland seniors can trust

As a former legislator, a nurse and a health care policy expert, I've been the advocate for your needs.

PROVEN RECORD OF RESULTS – sponsoring, voting and working for...

- Protecting benefits for seniors
- A program to screen for breast cancer and other preventive measures for nursing home residents
- Day care for medically handicapped seniors
- A Hospice Commission
- Advocate for insurance coverage for prescription drugs and home health care
- Advocate for neighborhood safety – community policing, stricter gun control and stronger victim's rights

AWARDS INCLUDE:

Maryland Public Health Association Legislator of the Year

Home Health Care Award

George and Tess Hurwitz Award, Hebrew Home of Greater Washington – for contributions to senior citizens and the community

Campaign materials reprinted courtesy of Marilyn Goldwater, Maryland State House of Delegates.

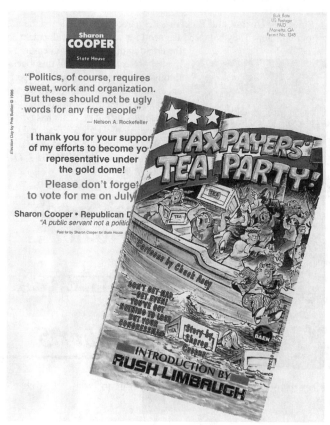

Campaign materials reprinted courtesy of Sharon Cooper, Georgia State Representative.

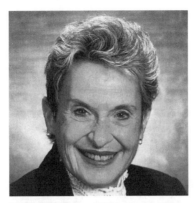

Paula Hollinger, Maryland State Senator.

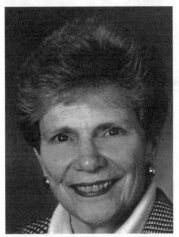

Patricia Vance, Pennsylvania State Representative.

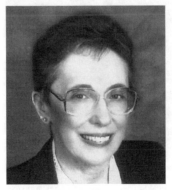

Marilyn Lee, Hawaii State Representative.

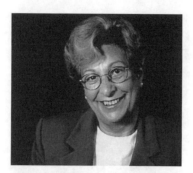

Marilyn Goldwater, Maryland State House of Delegates.

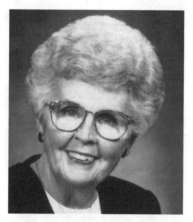

Beverly Nelson, Iowa State Representative.

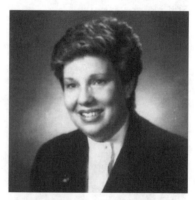

Muriel Shore, Fairfield City Mayor.

Is This a Job Worth Fighting (Fair) For?

Mom was elected—despite her opponent's tactics. Will negative campaigns discourage others?

By ANGELA UHERBELAU

FIVE MONTHS AGO I WALKED into my mother's house on a rainy afternoon. She was sitting on the couch, shoulders slumped forward, holding an oversized piece of mail. She looked at me, dejected, and asked, "Why do I put myself through this?"

My mom's an elected state representative from southern Oregon. The flier she held in her hand had arrived in her mailbox just that morning. It was a so-called hit piece put out by her opponent. Ugly in tone, it painted several of Mom's votes as being anti-education. The most inflammatory part of the piece cited no source and read: "After Judy Uherbelau's four years in Salem, kids face more danger from drugs and violence in school than ever."

To you voters out there who have seen much worse in your own mailbox, a charge like this may strike you as tame. To an exhausted candidate who lives in a small town of 19,000, however, it can be devastating. Who wants to walk into the local grocery store or library and wonder, "Do people here believe those awful things about me? Do they believe that my service in the Oregon Legislature has been harmful to kids?"

To make matters worse, days earlier Mom's opponent had said in a television interview, "Judy seems to care more about lawsuits than compassion." Considering my mother's background, this statement was almost comical. Mom spent 15 years as a registered nurse, including four as a Peace Corps volunteer in the Mariana Islands. In southern Oregon, she started a theater program in nursing homes, helped develop the county's first AIDS task force and established a teen-health clinic at our local high school. But not all voters were aware of Mom's history—a fact her opponent was banking on.

The sound bite referred to a vote on a Good Samaritan bill which would have exempted lay persons who aid accident victims from legal prosecution, unless they were proved grossly negligent. While Oregon law already covered those with medical training, the 1997 Oregon House of Repre-

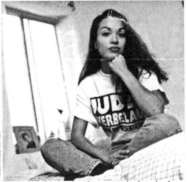

'After a while, people subconsciously slam the door on the idea of entering public service themselves'

sentatives considered exempting everyone, whether they had training or not. Mom was the only representative to vote against it. Her reason: as a registered nurse, she had seen patients suffer irreversible spinal injuries from being improperly moved following an accident. While she agreed that everyone should be encouraged to stop and comfort an accident victim (as well as call for the appropriate emergency assistance), she didn't believe untrained people should attempt to administer medical care. Mom's opponent tried to turn this conscientious vote into a callous one.

Some may say that being Judy's daugh-

ter makes me unable to judge fairly any challenge to her ability as a legislator. I expect her opponent to take issue with her legislative record in order to point out clear differences between them. What I object to is having her record distorted to fit a sound bite or her entire life history twisted into a catch phrase.

When a race occurs on the national or even state level, we voters tend to depersonalize it. From such a distance, the candidates seem more like actors than flesh and blood. Campaigns take on epic proportions, with each contender trying to paint himself or herself as Moses and the opponent as Pharaoh.

While such dramatization may stir voters enough to get them to cast ballots in presidential and statewide races, it can do more harm than good on the local level. Who wants to run for an often-unpaid, unglamorous seat on the city council when there's always that hit piece or dark sound bite waiting in the wings? After a while, people subconsciously slam the door on the idea of entering public service themselves.

It's tempting to throw up our hands and say "Politics is a dirty business," but I think that we Americans have more influence over campaigns than we know. In Mom's case, the tide began to turn when many supporters wrote letters to the newspapers condemning negative tactics and pointing out Mom's strengths as a legislator. A local group of voters organized a protest, calling on her opponent to run a clean campaign. In endorsing Mom, all the local papers called attention to her opponent's willingness to distort her record.

I must confess that when I saw my mother so discouraged five months ago, my first instinct was to see what dirt we could dig up on her opponent. Mom was much wiser than I and chose to finish the race the way she began it: cleanly. Voters responded by giving her a 12 percentage-point victory, the largest margin the seat had seen in something like 20 years.

Due to term limits, the 1999 Oregon legislative session will be Mom's last. Her opponent, however, is expected to run again in the year 2000. I hope that both she, and whoever runs against her, will choose to run a clean and accurate campaign. We Americans face too many critical issues for our candidates to spend their time—and ours—on much less.

Uherbelau works for the California Democratic Party and is pursuing an acting career.

Index